HEART HEALTHY COOKBOOK FOR BEGINNER

The ultimate guide for heart health with 1200 days of low-sodium, low-fat recipes and a 30-day meal plan.

GRACE RUIZ

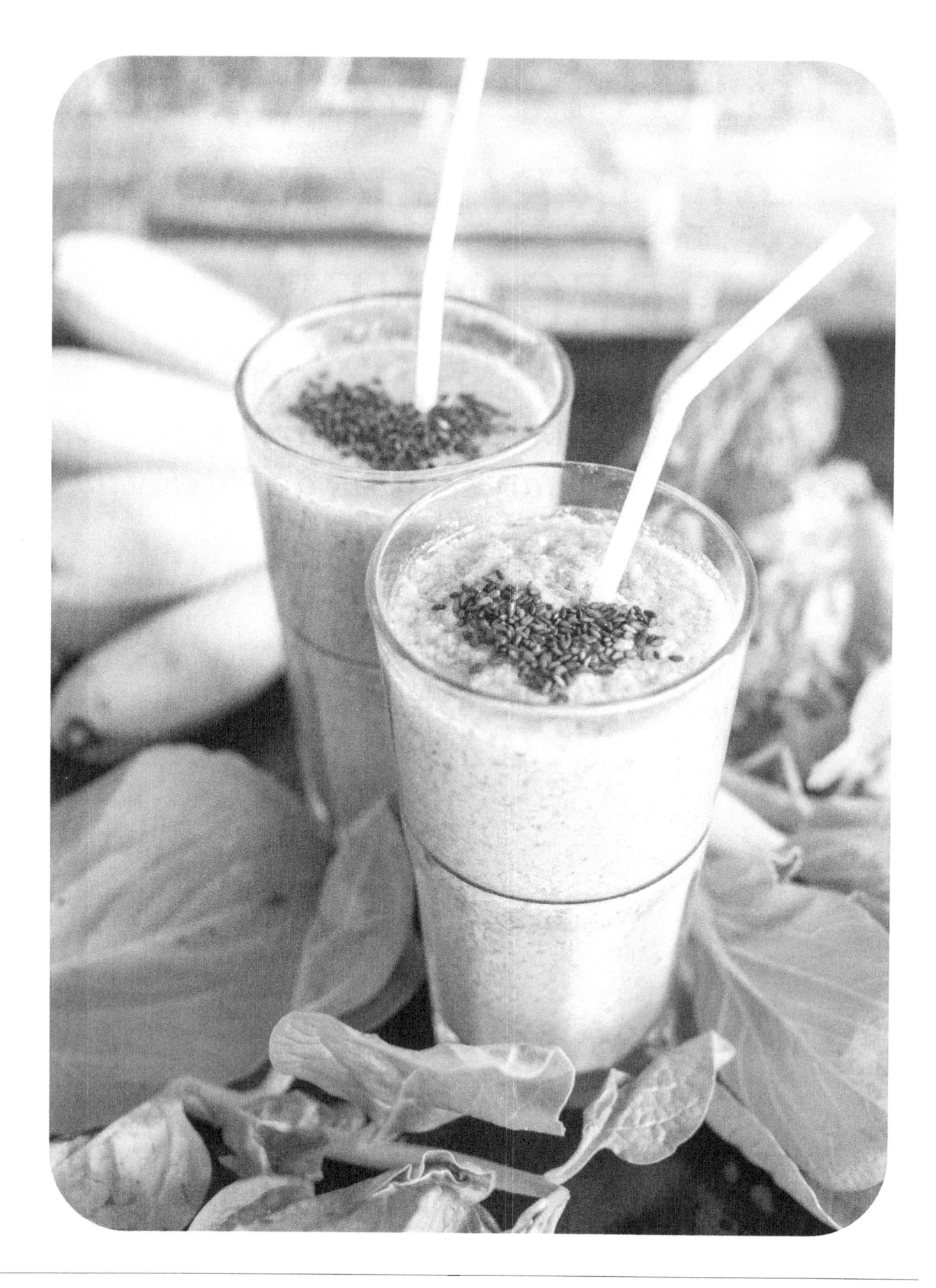

© **Copyright 2022 by Grace Ruiz - All rights reserved.**

This document is geared towards providing exact and reliable information in regard to the topic and issue covered. The publication is sold with the idea that the publisher is not required to render accounting, officially permitted, or otherwise, qualified services. If advice is necessary, legal or professional, a practiced individual in the profession should be ordered.

- From a Declaration of Principles, which was accepted and approved equally by a Committee of the American Bar Association and a Committee of Publishers and Associations.

In no way is it legal to reproduce, duplicate, or transmit any part of this document in either electronic means or in printed format. Recording of this publication is strictly prohibited, and any storage of this document is not allowed unless with written permission from the publisher. All rights reserved.

The information provided herein is stated to be truthful and consistent, in that any liability, in terms of inattention or otherwise, by any usage or abuse of any policies, processes, or directions contained within is the solitary and utter responsibility of the recipient reader. Under no circumstances will any legal responsibility or blame be held against the publisher for any reparation, damages, or monetary loss due to the information herein, either directly or indirectly.

Respective authors own all copyrights not held by the publisher.

The information herein is offered for informational purposes solely and is universal as so. The presentation of the information is without contract or any type of guaranteed assurance.

The trademarks that are used are without any consent, and the publication of the trademark is without permission or backing by the trademark owner. All trademarks and brands within this book are for clarifying purposes only and are owned by the owners themselves, not affiliated with this document.

Table of content

INTRODUCTION 10

CHAPTER 1: THE BASIC PRINCIPLES OF THE HEART-HEALTHY DIET 12
- WHAT IS MEANT BY HEALTHY EATING AND CARING FOR THE HEART? 12
- THE GOOD AND THE BAD FATS 13
- ALCOHOL 13
- THE FRENCH PARADOX 14
- EXCESS OF CALORIES 14
- EATING HABITS 15
- THE ROLE OF OBESITY ON OUR HEART 15
- HOW TO GRADUALLY REDUCE EXCESS CALORIES 16

CHAPTER 2: WHAT ARE THE RISK FACTORS FOR HEART DISEASE? 19
- THE ROLE OF NUTRITION 20

CHAPTER 3: FOODS TO EAT AND TO AVOID 22
- FOOD TO EAT 22
- FOOD TO AVOID 23

CHAPTER 4: RECOMMENDATIONS OF THE AMERICAN HEART ASSOCIATION (AHA) 25
- BEWARE OF THE HEAT 25
- HYDRATE YOUR BODY 27
- CHECK THE MEDICATIONS YOU ARE TAKING 27
- PLAY SPORTS 28
- DON'T FORGET YOUR SOCIAL RELATIONSHIPS. 28

CHAPTER 5: BREAKFAST RECIPES 30
- CHEESE AND VEGETABLE FRITTATA 31
- QUINOA WITH CINNAMON AND PEACHES 31
- PANCAKES MULTIGRAIN WITH STRAWBERRY SAUCE 31
- BOWL OF GUACAMOLE AND MANGO WITH BLACK BEANS 32
- CHOCOLATE BANANA OATS 32
- HOMEMADE GRANOLA 32
- NUTRITIOUS BAGELS 32
- BREAKFAST OATMEAL 33
- BANANA OATMEAL CUPS 33
- PEANUT BUTTER OATS 33
- BREAKFAST PIZZA 33
- BREAKFAST WRAPS 34
- PORTOBELLO MUSHROOMS FLORENTINE 34
- PEANUT BUTTER OATMEAL 34
- CHIA SEED PARFAITS 35

BREAKFAST TACOS 35
SPRING VEGETABLE FRITTATA 35
QUICHE WITH ASPARAGUS, SALMON, AND TOMATO 36
SAUSAGE AND EGG SANDWICH 36
TOMATO EGG TART 36
SPINACH WRAPS 37
VEGETABLE SHAKE 37
CASHEW NUT SHAKE 37
HUMMUS AND DATE BAGEL 37
CURRY TOFU SCRAMBLE 38
BREAKFAST SPLITS 38
TOMATO BASIL BRUSCHETTA 38
CREAMED RICE 38
EGG FOO YOUNG 39
CRANBERRY HOTCAKES 39

CHAPTER 6: LUNCH RECIPES 40

TURKEY KEEMA CURRY 41
ORZO, BEAN, AND TUNA SALAD 41
SMOKED HADDOCK AND SPINACH RYE TOASTS 41
CHIPOTLE CHICKEN LUNCH WRAP 41
SALMON WITH MARINADE 42
BALSAMIC ROAST CHICKEN 42
SALAD WITH BALSAMIC VINAIGRETTE 42
BEEF AND VEGETABLE KEBABS 42
BEEF AND VEGETABLE STEW 43
BEEF BRISKET 43
CARIBBEAN GRILLED PORK 43
DEEP, DARK, AND STOUT CHILI 44
GRILLED SHRIMP TACOS 44
CHICKEN SALAD SANDWICH 44
QUINOA BOWLS WITH SHRIMP 45
TOMATO WITH GARLICKY CHIVES 45
PEPPERED CHEESE WITH STOCKY CAULIFLOWER SOUP 45
PARSLEY CHICKPEA BOWLS WITH LEMON 45
TOMATO WITH CHEESY EGGPLANT SANDWICHES 46
LEMONY SALMON WITH SPICY ASPARAGUS 46
HALIBUT WITH LIME AND GINGER 46
LENTILS & RICE 47
CANNELLINI BEAN PIZZA 47
GARBANZO BEAN CURRY 47
POTATO SALAD 48
SPINACH BERRY SALAD 48
HEALTHY MINESTRONE 48
QUINOA VEGETABLE SOUP 49
GERMAN POTATO SOUP 49
PASTA PRIMAVERA 49

CHAPTER 7: DINNER RECIPES 51

SMOKY HAWAIIAN PORK 52

Chipotle Tacos 52
Zesty Pepper Beef 52
Italian Roast 52
Yummy Steak Bites 52
Teff with Broccoli Pesto 53
Warm Barley Salad with Spring Veggies 53
Roasted Shrimp and Veggies 53
Shrimp and Pineapple Lettuce Wraps 54
Grilled Scallops with Gremolata 54
Healthy Paella 54
Baked Pork Chops 55
Shish Kabob 55
Spicy Veal Roast 55
Barbecued Chicken 56
Barbecued Chicken-Spicy 56
Glazed Meatloaf 56
Chicken with Tarragon and Lentils, Pan-Roasted 56
Chicken with Lemon Pepper and Garlic 57
Teriyaki Chicken with Black Rice and Vegetables 57
Sweet and Sour Chicken with Rice 57
Pasta with Vegetables 58
Pumpkin Pasta Sauce 58
Vegan Bowl 58
Halibut with Tomato Salsa 59
Herb-Crust Cod 59
Honey Crusted Chicken 59
Zucchini-Chickpea Burgers 59
Chicken Tenders with Bagel Seasoning 60
Honey-Garlic Chicken Thighs 60

CHAPTER 8: MEAT RECIPES 61

Spiced Beef 62
Tomato Beef 62
Beef Tenderloin Medallions With Yogurt Sauce 62
Mustardy Zucchini Beef Burger 62
Garlicky Beef Tenderloin with Artichoke 63
Beef with Spicy Vegetable Stir-Fry 63
Beef Tenderloin with Balsamic Tomatoes 63
Fajita-Style Beef Tacos 64
One-Pot Spinach Beef Soup 64
Sesame Beef Skewers 64
Best Lasagna Soup 65

CHAPTER 9: FISH AND SEAFOOD RECIPES 66

Catfish with Egg Pecans 67
Roast Salmon with Tarragon 67
Pasta with Lemon Spiced Shrimp and Cheese 67
Tomatoes with Tilapia Tacos 67
Garlic-Baked Flounder 68
Seafood Dip 68

Spinach Shrimp Alfredo 68
Shrimp Scampi 68
Fish Salad 69
Flavors Shrimp Scampi 69
Creamy Tuna Salad 69
Citrus Tilapia 69
Lebanese-style cod fillets 70
Salmon Sage Bake 70
Pine Nut Haddock 70
Catalán Salmon Tacos 70
Salmon with Farro Pilaf 71
Salmon and Cauliflower Sheet Pan 71
Spicy Trout Sheet 71
Salmon Patties 72

CHAPTER 10: POULTRY RECIPES 73

Garlicky Chicken Thighs with Vinegar 74
Zesty Chicken Kebabs with Eggplants 74
Spaghetti with Chicken Meatballs 74
Chicken Fajitas with Mango Salsa 75
Peppered Chicken Tortilla Casserole 75
White Chicken Chili 75
Parmesan Chicken Cutlets 76
Chicken Quesadillas 76
Copycat Olive Garden Chicken Gnocchi Soup 77
Lemon Pepper Chicken 77

CHAPTER 11: VEGETARIAN MAIN COURSE RECIPES 78

Zucchini with Cheesy Lasagna 79
Celery with Mushroom Bolognese 79
Chili Bean Mix with Scallion 79
Cheese crepes with spinach 80
Creamy Vegetable Quiche 80
Cannellini Bean Pizza 81
Garbanzo Bean Curry 81
Pinto Bean Tortilla 81
Green frittata 82
Lemon Chicken Orzo Soup 82
Spiced eggplant fritters 82
Broccoli Rice Casserole 83
Grilled Eggplant and Tomato Pasta 83
Potato and Vegetable Casserole 83
Cereal bowl with cashew and tahini sauce 83
Creamy Zucchini And Potato Soup 84
Vegan Ratatouille 84
Homemade Rice Pilaf 84
Fried Rice Tom Yum 85
Healthy banana cookies with oatmeal 85

CHAPTER 12: SNACK RECIPES 87

Hummus 88
Honey-Lime Berry Salad 88
Whipped Ricotta Toast 88
Sikil Peak (Pumpkin Seed Salsa) 88
Sweet Potato Hummus 89
Spiced Chickpeas with Peppered Parsley 89
Roasted Plums with Honey-Yogurt Sauce 90
Garlic Popcorn 90
Zucchini Pizza Bites 90
Tangy green beans 90
Corn pudding 90
Chili-Lime Grilled Pineapple 91
Baked Bell Peppers 91
Citrus Asparagus 91
Lemon Brussels Sprouts 91

CHAPTER 13: SMOOTHIE AND JUICE 92

Jalapeño with Cilantro Juice 93
Grapy Weight Loss Juice 93
Icy Orange Juice with Lemon 93
Fruity Mixed Juice 93
Avocado Mix with Ice 93
Apple-Carrot Juice 93
Cinnamon with Potatoes Juice 94
Mint lime with cucumber and carrot 94
Kale-Banana smoothie 94
Apple Tart smoothie 94
Kiwi, Zucchini, and Pear smoothie 94
Green Mango smoothie 95
Carroty Breakfast Grind 95
Juicy Morning Blaster 95
Fresh Morning Juice 95
Early-Berry Juice 95
Rise and Shine Morning Juice 95
Green Monster 96
Orange Sunrise 96
Purple Passion 96

CHAPTER 14: DESSERT 97

Apricot Crisp 98
Baked Apples with Almonds 98
Berries with Balsamic Vinegar 98
Cookie Cream Shake 98
Creamy Fruit Dessert 98
Cheddar Cake 99
Yogurt Cheesecake 99
Sweet potato and pumpkin pie 99
Crepes with strawberries and cream cheese 99
Apple-Berry Cobbler 100
Mint chocolate dessert with banana 100

- Baked Apples with Cherries and Almonds 100
- Fruit Cake 101
- Carrot cookies 101
- Hot chocolate pudding 101
- Roasted plums with walnut crumble 102
- Mascarpone and honey figs 102
- Chocolate "Mousse" with Greek Yogurt and Berries 102
- Meringues with Strawberries, Mint, and Toasted Coconut 102
- Pistachio-Stuffed Dates 103

CONVERSION TABLES OF THE VARIOUS UNITS OF MEASUREMENT 104
30 DAY MEAL PLAN 105
CONCLUSION 108

introduction

The heart is one of our body's most essential and vital organs. Its health profoundly affects our life and everything that revolves around us.

The heart is muscular in all respects, and its nature is involuntary, meaning it is impossible to control its beats and range at all. You can check.

Today in an increasingly awake society, which never stops and always has very intense rhythms. But, of course, I am not referring only to our professional or working life but also to our family life, our loved ones, and our entertainment. Therefore, keeping up with everything becomes more and more complicated, and we often tend to sacrifice our health to satisfy other social or professional commitments.

When we are young, our body has a very efficient ability to adapt and respond. Consequently, micro-signals or impulses of some warning are not perceived or seen as a minimum thing. However, with the passage of time and with aging, our body reduces its efficiency and ability to respond to any form of stress, and we are always affected by it.

Is it possible to take care of your heart actively?

The answer to this complex question is yes, and, given recent studies, it is possible to significantly improve the nature and health of your heart, starting with your diet.

That's right, nutrition has been shown to play a central and decisive role in the health of your heart.

Knowing about healthy food and foods that are good for your heart is the foundation for restoring your metabolism and overall heart health.

As we said at the beginning, the heart is a muscle and should be treated. For example, those who practice intense sporting activity and a competitive level such as tennis know how important it is to have strong arm muscles that can withstand severe stress. But at the same time, having resistant and robust arm muscles are useless if the legs and lungs are not trained. So, taking care of your heart is essential, but you don't have to focus only on this aspect, but on all the things in your life.

It is necessary to make a local mind, that is, to understand which are stress factors, toxic, that must be eliminated, or the heart replaced with the positive aspects that restore the health of your heart. The human body is an extraordinary natural machine capable of withstanding severe stress and self-healing. It is up to us to take the right and corrective actions to take to bring our body in general to its ideal shape and health.

Food, therefore, plays a central role in your health and heart. Thanks to this book, you will discover which are all the foods that can bring a benefit in the concise and long term to your heart. Still, you will also find out the good practices to keep your heart active and how to improve its performance.

Your physical condition is, therefore, the central element of the result. The more tired, sore, and overweight we are, the more complex our heart health will be restored.

For this reason, I recommend contacting a specialist doctor who can provide you with a more specific overview of what lies behind physical and mental well-being. But for now, let's focus on the nature of the delicious food and dishes you can prepare to make your heart feel better.

Enjoy the reading

Chapter 1: the basic principles of the heart-healthy diet

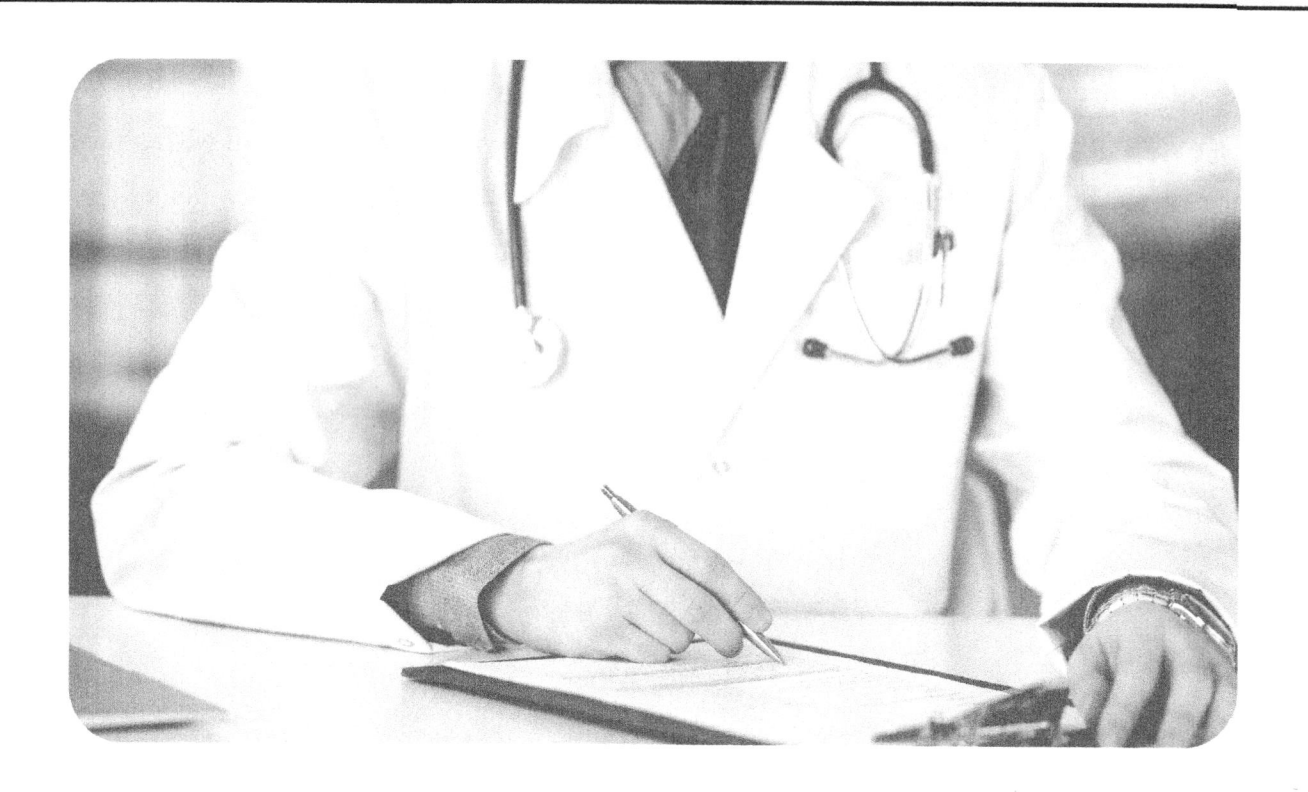

What is meant by healthy eating and caring for the heart?

Healthy eating is a diet or nourishment that helps your body eliminate toxic substances, restores metabolism efficiency, and makes you feel good. To eat correctly, it is, therefore, necessary to know the benefits that foods or ingredients in your diet bring to your heart and your body.

The food is delicious and flavorful when we eat out in restaurants or our fast-food joints. Unfortunately, these fabulous flavors hide inside various ingredients and chemicals that, in the long run, can cause severe problems of all kinds to our bodies. In fact, the first piece of advice I would like to give you is not to go often too fast-food restaurants or places where the ingredients used are not precise. Cooking at home can sometimes be difficult and time-consuming. However, I can assure you that if you have a particular purpose, to take care of your person, cooking will become a pleasure and fun. Furthermore, all the recipes in this book are straightforward to make, and you don't need a lot of experience.

So, the first thing you need to consider is healthy food. What is healthy food? Healthy food is food that is good for your heart, and that is beneficial.

The good and the bad fats

Not all fats are created equal, and not all fats are toxic. In our diet, we should range and vary the foods we eat every day and try to diversify. It would also be enough to follow the seasonality of some foods or ingredients to correctly change our diet according to the climate and the territory in which we live.

The fats we can classify as our friends are generally unsaturated or polyunsaturated fats and are found in many vegetables, dried fruit (nuts), and fish, incredibly fresh and non-canned.

On the other hand, toxic fats are mainly found in red meat, sweets, and all high-calorie foods. Our body does not need these substances and does not eliminate them; instead, it accumulates them.

We often think that eating fat is wrong and should be avoided. But, in fact, many fats, especially those of vegetable origin or some facts contained in some fish, promote a healthy and positive lifestyle.

It is, therefore, good to know which foods contain these substances and start consuming them. This book will find many health-promoting recipes with this type of fat.

Alcohol

Alcohol is food in all respects and is usually taken in drinks or mixed drinks (cocktails). However, little-known information is the number of calories that alcohol supplies to our bodies. Briefly, if carbohydrates provide 4 kcal, proteins 6 kcal, and fats 9 kcal, do you know how many kcal alcohols offer when taken? The answer is shocking, which is almost 9 kcal, which is a value similar to fat.

The human body is capable of metabolizing fats, carbohydrates, and proteins. But unfortunately, it is unable to metabolize alcohol; in fact, this is immediately excreted in the urine. Alcohol belongs to the category of bad fats.

However, suppose the total amount in the body begins to be high. In that case, our body, in particular the kidneys first and the heart after, start to no longer work properly, and alcohol literally destroys the metabolism.

So, pay attention to the use of alcohol and limit or eliminate its presence in your diet.

If you really can't do without it, try to take it in small quantities next to meals; this way, with active digestion, the body will have better efficiency for its expulsion.

The French paradox

France is the land of beautiful cuisine and delicious dishes that are beautiful to look at. The French, however, have a minor flaw; that is, they love to eat cheeses of all types and tastes at any time of the meal, both as an aperitif and as an accompaniment to the first meal or as a second course or even as desserts. Cheeses are mainly rich in fats and proteins.

So, the question that arises spontaneously is: How do the French take all these fats (through cheeses) and not have many heart diseases or others related to metabolism?

The answer that many experts have given themselves by analyzing French cuisine and, above all, the eating habits of the subjects studied is truly surprising. Generally speaking, every French family has a vast knowledge of the culture of wine (a drink that contains alcohol) and therefore does not hold back in its daily consumption. Attention the consumption of wine in France is among the highest in Europe. Still, every family does not exaggerate their consumption; somewhat, it limits itself to a small glass after a meal.

A small amount of alcohol after a meal, in some cases, can help blood circulation as alcohol also can slightly elasticize the capillaries where the blood flows; therefore, more blood reaches the digestive system, and fats and proteins (present in cheeses) are metabolized with greater efficiency.

France can be an excellent example of how to regularly consume a very moderate amount of wine (not a super alcoholic) and still stay fit.

My general advice is to go to your doctor and see what he recommends and what information he can give you about alcohol. Also, if you take certain drugs or therapies, alcohol can harm these or other drug treatments. So, before you start a new habit, get yourself informed.

Excess of calories

Make food your medicine and your medicine your food (Hippocrates)

Eating is a pleasure, and, in some respects, it can also be a moment of conviviality. Every single food, chemical, and natural substance you ingest every day profoundly affects your heart's health. A strong and healthy heart is a heart that has consistently received healthy attention and food.

In many cases, it can be verified that our meal is full of energy and calories, i.e., the amount of energy that the meal provides is greater than the general energy expenditure of our day. This inevitably leads to weight gain and many other negative consequences.

Therefore, paying attention to the portions, you take and the available quantity of food you eat daily is the second step that must be taken to restore heart health.

Many doctors say we should get up from the table with a slight hunger to immediately burn all the food ingested.

I realize that this eating habit turns out to be complicated to implement, also because we often live in complex family situations.

So, start today to see how many high-calorie foods you eat daily and gradually reduce their consumption; also, try adding one or more servings of fruit and vegetables to each meal. This will also increase the amount of natural fiber in your diet.

In fact, fibers are your best allies for losing weight, restoring the good bacteria that live in your intestine, and, consequently, the health of your heart.

Eating habits

An essential aspect is also the eating habits you have.

In fact, being regular and having indicative times on when to eat your meals is very important first to regulate your metabolism and restore your heart's health.

One piece of advice I would like to give you is to write on your smartphone what your main meals of the week will be, what you would like to eat, and on what day; in this way, you will know how to best organize your meals, and you can even indulge yourself if, for example, you meet a friend or you want to go out and dine out.

Being organized is the best starting point to prepare your meals and start having healthy habits that will bring you many benefits in the short and long term.

Finally, try to avoid eating off-meal times or at times when it is not expected to eat. Even if not too caloric, these snacks kill the body's regular metabolism. Consequently, all the fundamental values of the heart are modified to make room for digestion and metabolism.

The role of obesity on our heart

Why doesn't obesity help our hearts?

Obesity is one of the most widespread diseases in our country; the data are alarming; they are proliferating and are extending even to the youngest; this means that there is no authentic culture about food, and many of the eating habits of our population are entirely wrong.

Body fat does not help blood circulation at all. Consequently, all blood vessels (such as arteries, veins, capillaries, etc.) are blocked by the presence of fat.

The heart of an obese subject is very stressed; this is because it has to pump several times, even in the resting phase and its range and efficiency are very low as the blood does not flow properly throughout the body.

Blood pressure is also too high, especially in moments of rest. Therefore, an obese person is a person who gets tired very quickly, even with small and straightforward efforts, precisely because the heart is always too active, and the blood pressure is too high.

Unfortunately, obese people often have other complications on a professional or social level and often find themselves alone with their problems. There is no magic pill or general medicine to treat obesity. Still, a structured and guided path with one or more experts is required.

How to gradually reduce excess calories

Reducing calories for the day is the right solution to most of your problems. But unfortunately, this turns out to be a very long and complex process, and it is not easy. But instead, it is necessary to build small habits that are healthy and healthy for your body and your heart. Above all, the benefits are not immediate but are seen in the long term. But I assure you that your life changes drastically once you get the results you were hoping for.

1. Start with simple walks. Walking is good for our blood circulation and our mood. In addition, walking involves slightly prolonged energy consumption. Therefore, it is forbidden to eat or nibble something when walking. This activates basal metabolism, which is the one that burns fat. Finally, I recommend that you take your walk in the company of a person who knows you well or in the company of music or audiobooks.

2. Involve your partner or a friend, or a person who has the same problem as you. Losing weight has never been easy, especially if you are alone. So, share your path and intentions with your loved ones, and don't be afraid of judgment. These people just want to help you, and they will be happy if you start losing weight and looking for the health of your body and heart.

3. Create a weekly healthy food menu. Correct eating habits should be installed as an APP on your smartphone. Therefore, having a series of healthy recipes that are good for your heart and your health is the right place to start creating your week's menu. If you find it

challenging to think about what to eat on any given day, start with the main meals first and then extend the rest of the planning to other meals and snacks.

4. Fill your agenda with things to do, even simple ones, so as not to think about food. Being busy and active always helps your brain to get distracted and not think about food. A "Do List" can be a valuable ally to fill the holes and free time of your day and consequently not think about food but instead do some positive activity that helps you lose weight.

5. I Prefer biking or walking in a car. The car is the most popular means of transport in our country and is also the most comfortable. However, if you can partially or entirely replace it with another means of transportation, don't think twice. For example, going to work by bike may seem embarrassing. Still, I assure you that the joy and well-being you feel when you arrive at your destination are priceless.

6. Don't be discouraged if you transgress. As I told you above, losing weight is not easy. You can often be fine for a week or 10 days but then fall back into the loop of old habits. This is because your body is changing and wants to eat high-calorie foods. In these situations, you don't have to get demoralized or depressed. Instead, you have to recognize your mistake and move on; that is, you have to try to find your own personal solution. For example, if you transgressed one Tuesday and ate a snack that you shouldn't have eaten, you can try eating an extra serving of fiber the next day. In this way, the feeling of satiety lasts up to a few more hours.

7. Talk about your new path to tons of people. That's right. If you have serious intentions to regain your health and guarantee your heart healthy and long life, share your thoughts and successes with everyone, even with social networks and with your loved ones. Go visit your friend and talk to him about what you are doing and what you want to achieve. All these actions have a positive effect on your mood and your serenity. Doing so also increases the chances of success.

8. Follow the advice of an expert. Industry experts are always intelligent, up-to-date, and have a lot of experience. Remember that these people follow tens or perhaps hundreds of patients and know exactly what is right and what is not. Do not follow the advice you find on the internet or social media; these are sometimes calibrated on the person writing and not your life. So, listen to the advice of a professional.

9. Join social groups at the gym, walking, and people who want to solve the same problems as you. Social networks (particularly Facebook) are an absolute gold mine that can help you thoroughly. Start following people who want to lose weight, people who have heart

problems, or people who have had intense experiences with it. Hear what they have to say and interact with them if you feel like it. The exchange of ideas and opinions will help you understand which is your best and healthy path and, in this way, recalibrate your goals in the best way.

Chapter 2: What are the risk factors for heart disease?

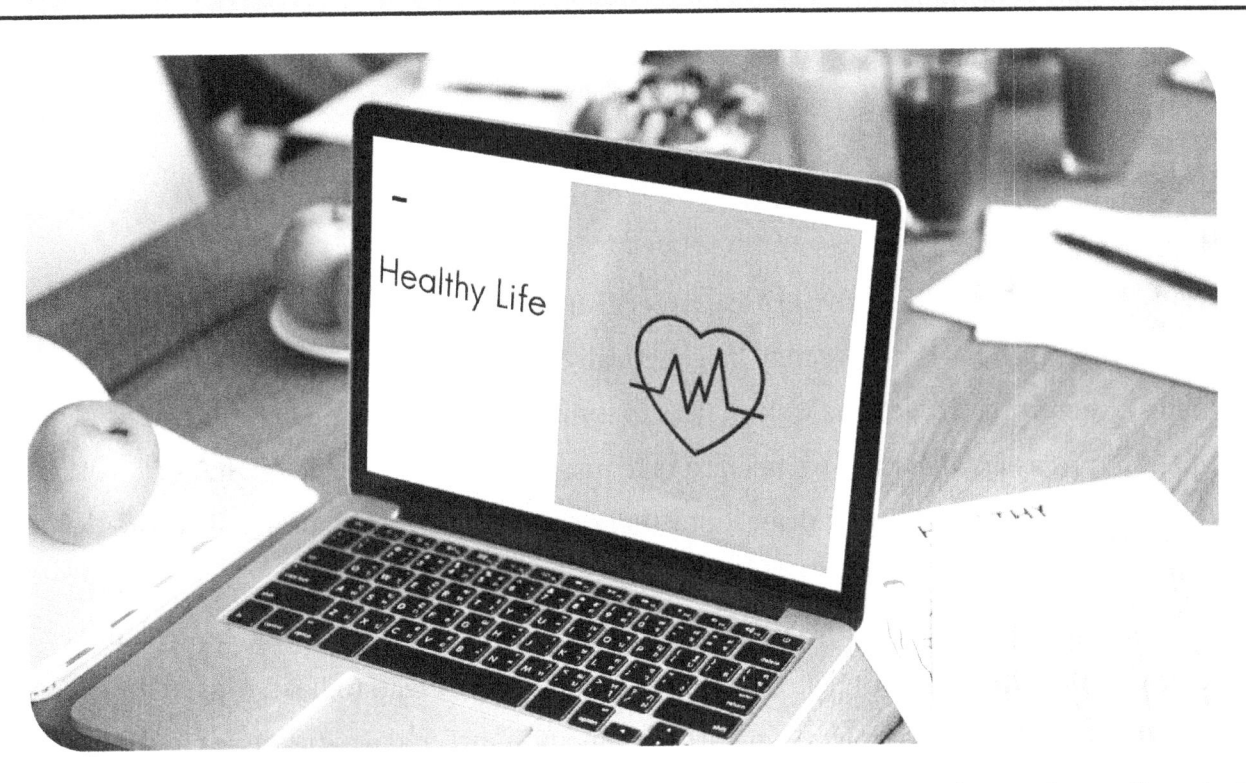

Here is a list of toxic habits that compromise your heart health. You must know them all as their prevention allows you to adopt relatively healthy habits and behaviors and eliminate or reduce the toxic ones.

Remember that in this list, you will find general indications. The negative effect triggered has been repeatedly demonstrated by many scientific studies that have studied healthy patients or patients with specific syndromes.

Knowing them is your second starting point to change and fix your heart.

The main risks that lead to heart problems are:

- obesity
- low physical activity
- Smoke
- Alcohol
- Stress
- Infectious diseases
- Sedentary lifestyle

- Chronic fatigue
- Diabetes
- Arrhythmias
- Metabolic syndrome
- Cholesterol too high
- Heart attack
- Excess salt

Analyzing this list thoroughly, two critical aspects are noted.

The first is that in some cases, we may be genetically predisposed to a given disease (such as type 1 diabetes); therefore, the actions we can take to limit this phenomenon are relatively few. For example, in the case of diabetes, we need to take insulin and monitor blood glucose levels. But there may also be other inherited diseases or those encountered accidentally on a trip or workplace.

The second aspect that we must necessarily consider is our general behavior. Some habits such as a sedentary lifestyle, smoking, alcohol, or obesity inevitably lead to heart-related or even more severe health-related diseases. Here you are we can and must make a difference in these situations. Changing a toxic habit is not easy, but neither is it impossible. Therefore, we must know the effects all these negative factors can cause on the heart and have a strategy to eliminate them immediately. The more time passes, the less we will have to stop it. Furthermore, these habits are acquired; they are not inherited. So, start looking for health now and eliminate anything that's not good for your heart and body.

The role of nutrition

A wrong diet produces toxic effects on the heart. The heart is a natural organ for our body, and we must necessarily take care of it for its proper functioning. Food and all-natural substances are our best allies (in addition to healthy habits such as playing sports and quitting smoking) to ensure the best functioning of the heart. Thanks to this splendid cookbook, you will find all the best dishes for your diet that you can easily share with your loved ones. You will also have the absolute certainty that everything you prepare is healthy and results from a lot of experience. Taking care of the heart does not mean being on a diet and eating only boiled and tasteless foods; in reality, you will find many recipes to satisfy all your tastes and other sensory organs, such as smell and sight. In addition, your diners will be amazed at how beautiful and relatively simple it is to prepare healthy food.

Finally, remember that each recipe has been designed to keep your heart in the best of its state. As a result, you will no longer have to worry about looking for hidden or unknown ingredients in junk food packages.

The natural substances contained in dried fruit, vegetables, legumes, and vegetables generally have extraordinary powers. Their intake should be daily, and we should never forget to take them; they should become an integral part of your diet. The benefits you will discover will be visible in the long run, but the mood of your days will change quickly.

Chapter 3: Foods to eat and to avoid

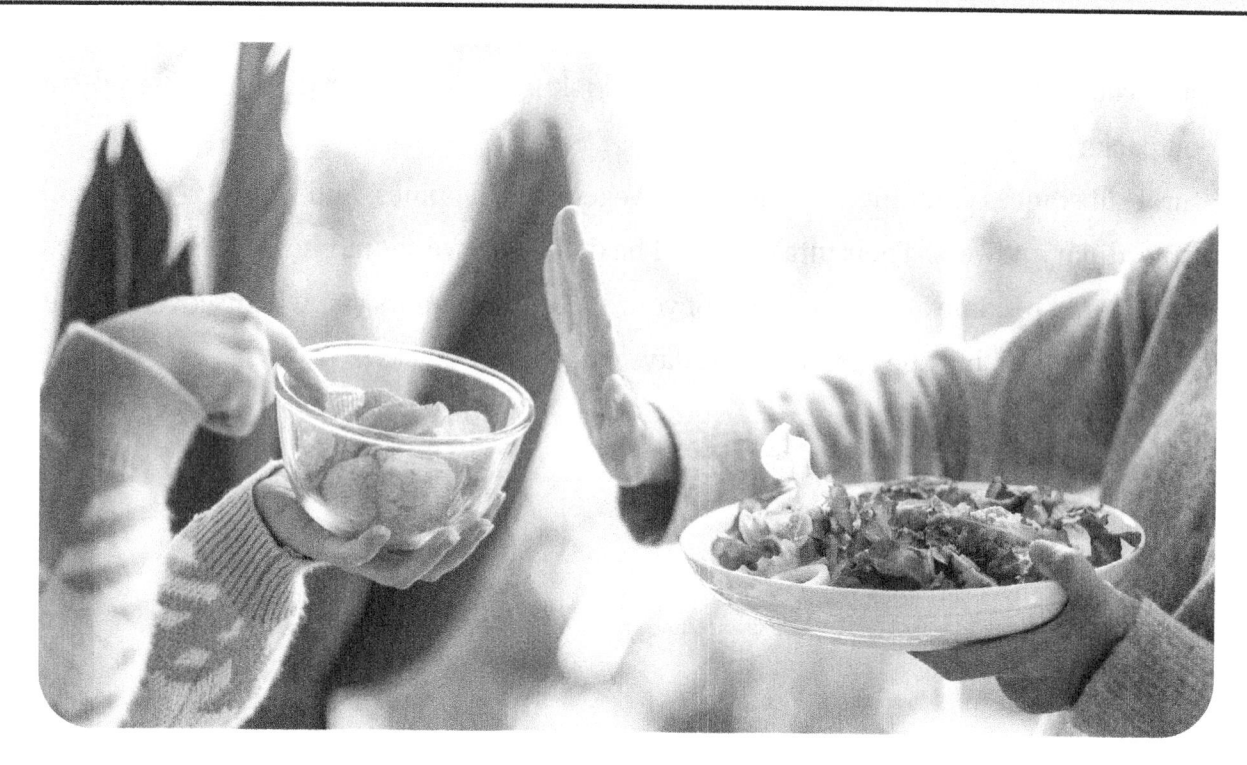

In this chapter, we see which are the best foods that help and strengthen the overall health of your heart. They often contain vitamins, polyphenols, or simple natural substances that are good for your kindness and health. Remember never to overdo their intake but rather try to vary the dishes with more healthy foods rather than focusing only on one type of ingredient.

Food to eat

- Asparagus
- Beans
- Peas
- Chickpeas
- Lentils
- Red berries
- Blackberries
- Broccoli
- Cabbage
- Chia seeds

- Flax seed
- Dark chocolate> 75% in small doses
- Fish
- Fatty acids with high omega-3 content
- Green tea
- Tender
- Nuts
- Almonds
- Chestnuts
- Cashew nuts
- Pistachio
- Oatmeal blush
- Red wine, in small doses
- Spinach
- Swiss chard
- Red tomatoes
- Yellow tomatoes
- Green leafy vegetables
- Raw vegetables
- Carrots

Food to Avoid

The intake of these foods or ingredients should be limited or significantly reduced. Try to hire them as little as possible and find a suitable replacement if you can.

- Butter
- Lard
- Fat sauce
- Red meats
- Fatty meats
- Fried food with oil
- Canned meats

- Over-processed meats
- Cutlet
- Sweets bought
- Excess sugar
- French fries
- Ice creams
- Savory pies
- Sweet cakes
- Mayonnaise
- Ketchup
- BBQ sauce
- Spicy sauces
- Sweet sauces
- Vinegar
- Excess salt
- Packaged food

Chapter 4: Recommendations of the American Heart Association (AHA)

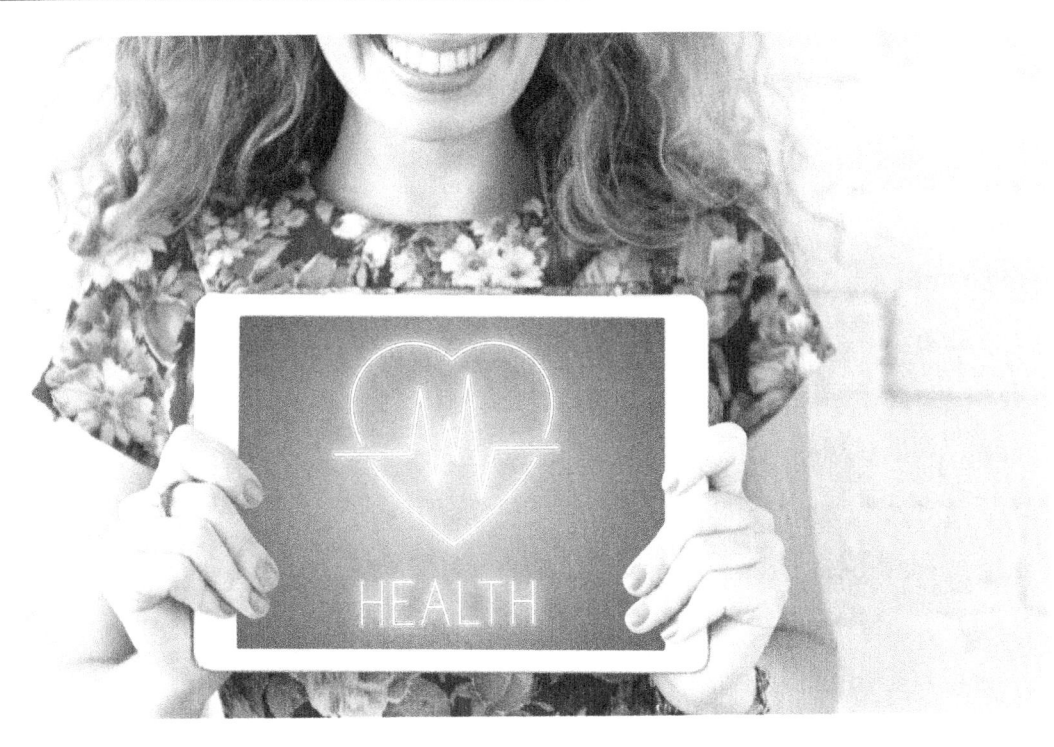

The AHA is an association studying people with heart problems for years. Their vast experience is involved in spreading clear and easy-to-interpret messages.

It is, therefore, suitable to know what they have seen and are studying. So often, they are the pioneers in providing simple guidance, but that can make a real difference.

Beware of the heat

A study recently published in "Circulation" that studied the number of average daily deaths in the hottest months of our country was reviewed and published. It has been found that when the average daily temperature reaches around 109 ° F, the average number of deaths of people suffering from heart disease doubles.

Often the precautions we take against heat are not enough, or we underestimate them.

In fact, heat is a risk factor and can also cause stroke in sensitive individuals.

So, if you are a person who has had a stroke, or you are overweight and not physically active, or if you have had cardiovascular disease, you need to take some simple but life-saving actions. Here are some of them:

- Do not go out during the hottest hours of the day
- Dress appropriately for higher temperatures
- Drink and hydrate your body
- Take regular breaks
- Follow your doctor's directions

The symptoms that excess heat can cause and therefore should sound like an alarm bell are:
- Sudden headache or cephalalgia
- Heavy and uncontrolled sweating
- Cold skin, shivering when it is actually hot
- Dizziness and fainting
- Feeble pulse
- Rapid pulse
- Muscle cramps, mild or severe
- Wheezing and difficulty breathing
- Nausea vomiting in both

While you are doing an activity, you feel even one of these symptoms, the advice of all doctors is to stop, breathe and if you can, shelter from the scorching heat and find a shaded area. Hydrate your body, and if you feel like it after a few minutes, you can resume your activity while constantly monitoring your body's signals.

The AHA also provides practical advice on what is best to eat in these extreme and difficult-to-manage situations. Indeed, when the hottest months of the year approaches, we should always have these foods that can make a difference in our fridge or on hand. Here are some of them:
- Chilled or frozen fruit
- Homemade popsicles made from 100% fruit juice.
- Fruit smoothies
- Cold salads rich in vegetables, beans, legumes, and healthy fish such as albacore tuna or salmon
- Crispy, chilled raw vegetables such as cucumbers, carrots, or celery with a light, fresh sauce

- Cold sparkling water with a splash of 100% fruit juice or slices of citrus or cucumber

Hydrate your body

Hydration is one of the most critical aspects of the general health of the human body. In fact, we are made up of more than 75% water. Water performs all the metabolic functions within our body, and in addition, it allows all tissues to regenerate correctly.

It is, therefore, reasonable to keep a body constantly well hydrated, especially during hot and sultry days. Unfortunately, we often forget to drink due to intense work activities or simply fail to bring a bottle of water with us.

If you are at risk of heart disease, remember that drinking water is essential. In this way, you will also facilitate blood circulation within your body and better fight the heat or the heat.

Not all waters are the same. We often don't notice it, but water plays a vital role in all metabolic processes and weight loss. So, drinking healthy water helps restore your body's balance.

The main aspects of the waters that we should monitor are:

- Optimal pH value, usually slightly above 7
- Content in mineral salts
- Fixed residue, look for waters that have values below 100 micrograms per liter
- Phosphate content, our legislation is stringent on bottled water, while the correct parameters are not always respected for tap water

All this information can be found conveniently on the label.

In fact, my advice is to find a couple of waters that are good to the taste and to always choose that one. The advantages of bottled water rather than ordinary tap water also refer to the periodic checks that companies are required to carry out and to the product's final quality.

Check the medications you are taking

Taking medications for a cardio-sensitive person is another aspect to consider. Often their intake is delayed by a few hours from the exact moment they must be taken, or they are taken superficially. For example, if you have to take your aspirin with a glass of water, do not use wine or another drink for its intake.

If you realize that the total medications you are taking are too many and, therefore, it is difficult to manage them all, try asking your doctor if it is possible to eliminate some of them or to take them at a specific time of the day. Sometimes there may be situations where multiple drugs contain the same active ingredient. So, it is good to monitor the number of daily medications taken and the quality, i.e., what you are actually taking.

Play sports

"Those who regularly practice a sport live a happy and intense life." These were the first words of a recent study that appeared in one of the journals. Indeed, it is. Sport helps you feel good, stay in shape and enjoy excellent health. But remember, you don't find benefit in the single occasional performance but consistency.

So, it is good to regularly practice sports even at low intensity (such as walking or free swimming) but to practice it constantly and daily, rather than practicing sports a couple of times a month in an intense way. But paradoxically, if we practice sports at the wrong time and incorrectly, we only risk hurting ourselves or straining the muscle too much.

Therefore, remember that a simple walk is enough to keep blood circulation active and optimal pressure values. Experts suggest taking at least 10,000 steps a day, better away from meals, especially outdoors.

At your disposal there is a wide choice of sports you can practice, my advice is to practice several, and you shouldn't get tired of playing sports, but instead, you have to have fun and have fun. Find your ally or partner who wants to play sports with you. Today, through social media, you can find any company or group of people who are following the same path as you and have the same interests as you. So, contact these people or choose a close friend or partner and start playing sports.

You will soon realize how many benefits physical activity brings, in addition to health; you will better heal your human relationships and relationships with loved ones.

Don't underestimate this aspect.

Don't forget your social relationships.

Human relationships are significant. Being active, having interests (of any kind), seeking a constructive dialogue, inquiring with friends about the result of the favorite team, participating in forums, going out for an aperitif, etc. are all fundamental activities to establish a climate of serenity, trust and of health.

A recent study published in 2020 showed that by improving their relationship activities, normal individuals with mild heart disease reduced the likelihood of having a severe heart-related problem by 86%.

These aspects are extraordinary and must be known. But human relationships allow us to be happy, pushing us to do more sports, eat better, and feel good with others.

A single person has little interest in others and even in himself. But, on the other hand, a person full of company and vitality is interested in feeling good and in shape.

Chapter 5: BREAKFAST RECIPES

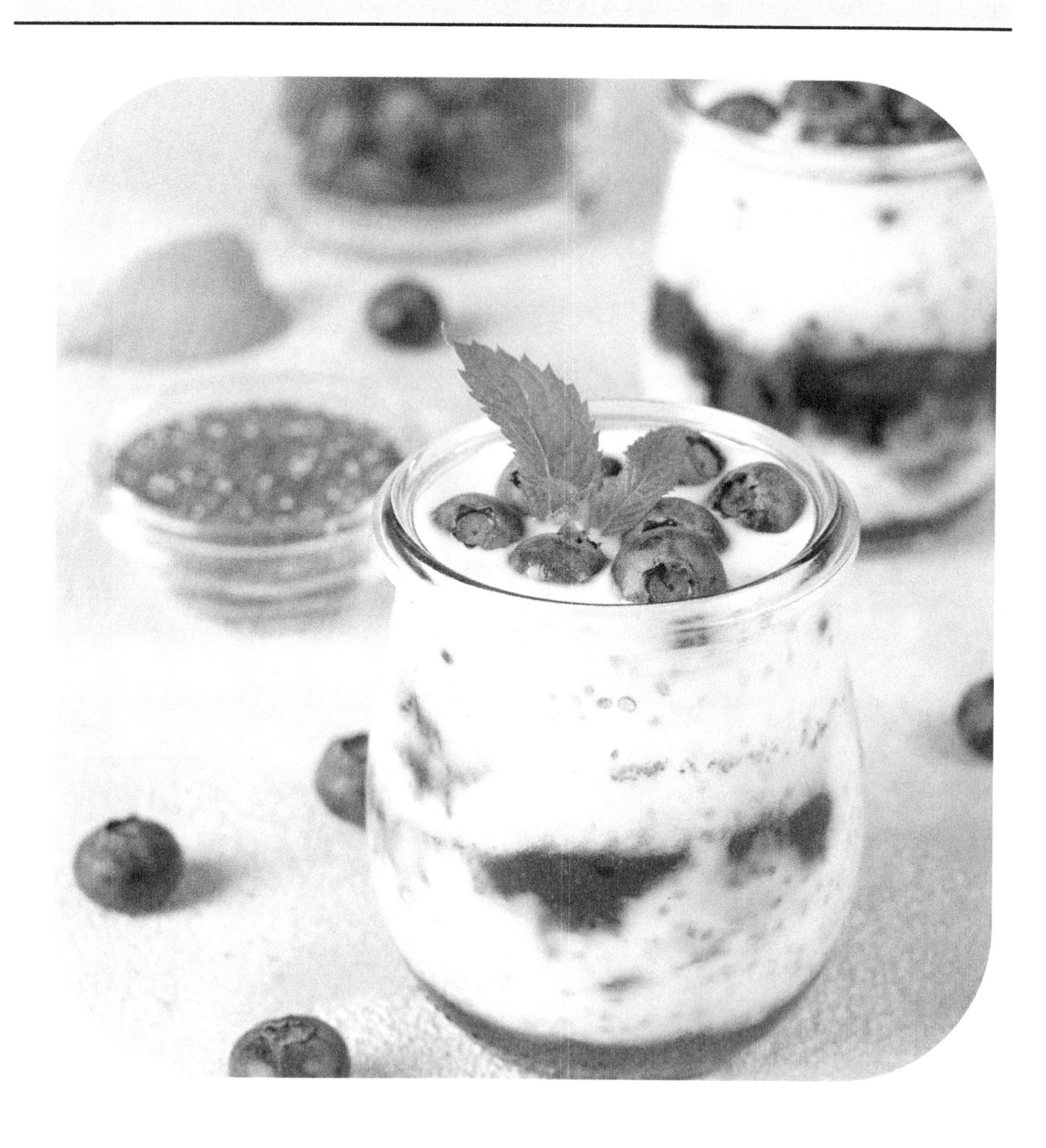

Cheese and Vegetable Frittata

Preparation time: 5 minutes **Cooking time:** 10 minutes **Servings:** 6
Ingredients:
- 6 eggs
- ⅓ cup mozzarella cheese (shredded)
- 2 tbsp. wheat flour
- 1 cup mushrooms
- 1 cup green bell pepper
- 2 tbsp. basil leaves
- 1 onion
- 1 cup frozen spinach
- 1 tsp. black pepper
- 1 clove garlic

Directions:
Preheat the oven. Beat the eggs in a bowl. Then, blend the pepper, wheat flour, and baking powder. Add the oil to the skillet over medium heat. Sauté in the onion for 3 minutes until soft. Add the basil and garlic and cook for a minute. Add the egg mixture and stir well to combine all the vegetables.
Sauté for minutes and add the shredded cheese. Place the pan in the oven and broil for 3 to 4 minutes. Once done, slice into pieces and serve.
Nutrition: Calories: 194 kcal | Fat: 7.8 g | Protein: 10 g | Carbs: 23 g | 28 mg Sodium

Quinoa with cinnamon and peaches

Preparation time: 5 minutes **Cooking time:** 1-hour **Servings:** 6
Ingredients:
- 2 tbsp. pecans
- 1 cup uncooked quinoa
- 2 cups water
- ¼ cup chopped pecans
- 2 cups frozen peach slices
- ½ tsp. cinnamon
- ¼ cup sugar
- 1 tsp. vanilla extract
- 1 cup fat-free half and half

Directions:
Spray the oil in the saucepan. Add the water, cinnamon, and quinoa. Cook over high heat until tender. Place the vanilla extract, sugar, and half and half in a bowl and mix well. Pour the quinoa into the bowl and add the peaches.
Serve and enjoy.
Nutrition: Calories: 254 kcal | Fat: 7 g | Protein: g | Carbs: 42 g | 47 mg Sodium

Pancakes Multigrain with Strawberry Sauce

Preparation time: 10 minutes **Cooking time:** 20 minutes **Servings:** 4
Ingredients:
- 1 cup strawberries
- ½ cup all-purpose white flour
- ¼ cup cornmeal
- 1 cup non-fat buttermilk
- ¼ cup apple juice
- ¼ cup wheat pastry
- 1 tbsp. canola oil
- 1 tbsp. baking powder
- 1 egg
- ¼ tsp. baking soda
- ¼ tsp. salt

Directions
Add the oil over the nonstick pan. Mix cornmeal and flour. Add the salt, baking powder, sugar, and baking soda. Whisk the egg in another bowl. Set in the canola oil and buttermilk. Blend the liquid and dry ingredients. Place the pan over the heat and place the batter in the skillet. Once pancakes cook from 1 side, flip them. Sauté until golden. Place the saucepan over the heat and add the apple and strawberries reserves. Once the sauce is ready, allow it to cool. And place them over the top of the muffins.
Nutrition: Calories: 409 kcal | Fat: 7 g | Protein: 8 g | Carbs: 81 g | 34 mg Sodium

Bowl of Guacamole and Mango with Black Beans

Preparation time: 10 minutes **Cooking time:** 0 minutes **Servings:** 2
Ingredients:
- 1 lime zest
- 1 lb black beans
- 1 small avocado
- 4 oz cherry
- 1 small mango
- ½ small pack of coriander
- 1 red onion

Directions:
Place all the ingredients in a bowl. Mix well and serve.
Nutrition: Calories: 341 kcal | Fat: 15 g | Protein: 11 g | Carbs: 33 g | 21 mg Sodium

Chocolate Banana Oats

Preparation time: 5 hours **Servings:** 1
Ingredients:
- ½ cup rolled oats
- ½ small banana
- 1 tbsp. chocolate hazelnut spread
- ½ cup water
- Salt

Directions:
Add salt, water, and oats to a bowl and mix them well.
Please place it in the fridge with a covered top. Top oats with chocolate hazelnut and sprinkle the salt over them. Serve and enjoy.
Nutrition: Calories: 303 kcal | Fat: 0.6 g | Protein: 6.6 g | Carbs: 52 g | 18 mg Sodium

Homemade Granola

Preparation time: 30 minutes **Cooking time:** 1 hour 30 minutes **Servings:** 20
Ingredients:
- 5 cups old-fashioned rolled oats
- 1 cup rice portions of cereal
- ¼ cup light brown sugar
- ⅓ cup pumpkin seeds roasted (unsalted pepitas)
- ¾ cup shredded coconut
- ¾ cup dried fruit
- ⅓ cup coarsely
- ⅓ cup slivered almond
- ⅓ cup honey
- 1 tbsp. ground cinnamon
- ⅓ cup canola oil
- ½ tsp. casher salt
- ½ tsp. vanilla extract
- 1 tsp. ginger
- ½ tsp. kosher salt

Directions:
Preheat the oven to 300°F. Mix all the dry ingredients in a bowl. Add all the remaining ingredients to the saucepan and set it to a simmer. Add all the dry ingredient mixture and mix them well. Place the oven and bake for half an hour, stirring continuously.
Serve and enjoy.
Nutrition: Calories: 215 kcal | Fat: 10.1 g | Protein: 3.9 g | Carbs: 29.9 g | 16 mg Sodium

Nutritious Bagels

Preparation time: 20 minutes **Cooking time:** 25 minutes **Servings:** 8
Ingredients:
- 2 cups wheat flour
- ¼ cup bread flour
- 2 tsp. yeast
- 2 tbsp. Honey
- ½ cup warm water
- ½ tbsp. olive oil
- 1 tbsp. vinegar

Directions:
Mix all the ingredients in the food processor. Prepare the flattened ball shape from the mixture. Make a hole in the ball to make a donut shape. Apply the oil to the foil and cover the donut in the sheet. Boil water

in the pan and boil in the ball one time. Remove from the sheet and bake for 25 minutes until brown.
Nutrition: Calories: 228.1 kcal | Fat: 3.7 g | Protein: 6.9 g | Carbs: 41.8 g | 22 mg sodium

Breakfast Oatmeal

Preparation time: 4 hours **Cooking time:** 0 minutes **Servings:** 8
Ingredients:
- 4 cups almond milk
- 1 tsp. cinnamon
- ⅓ cup raisins
- 2 packets of stevia
- 4 cups water
- ⅓ cup apricot
- 2 cups oats
- ⅓ cup cherries

Directions
Mix all the ingredients in a bowl. Cover the top and shake the bowl to mix the ingredients.
Serve in the breakfast.
Nutrition: Calories: 175.6 kcal | Fat: 3.2 g | Protein: 5.1 g | Carbs: 31.6 g | 25 mg sodium

Banana Oatmeal Cups

Preparation time: 10 mins **Cooking time:** 40 mins **Servings:** 4
Ingredients:
- 4 mashed bananas
- 2 eggs
- ½ tsp. salt
- 1½ c. low-fat milk
- 1 tsp. ground cinnamon
- 3 c. rolled oats
- ⅓ c. brown sugar
- 1 tsp. baking powder
- ½ c. chopped pecans
- 1 tsp. vanilla extract

Directions:
Preheat the oven to 375 ° Fahrenheit. Grease cupcake pans using cooking spray. Put salt, cinnamon, baking powder, vanilla, mashed bananas, milk, eggs, oats, and brown sugar in a bowl. Mix everything well using a spatula, then add the pecans and fold the mixture. Pour the mixture into the greased muffin dish until each compartment is about ¾ full. Bake for 30 minutes. Insert a toothpick into the middle of a muffin and then pull it out. If the toothpick comes out clean, the muffins are done. Cool muffins on a wire rack for ten minutes. You can also serve them when they are a little warm.
Nutrition: Calories 176; Fat 1.2g; Carbohydrates 26.4g; Proteins 5.2g; Cholesterol 33.4mg; Sodium 165.6mg; Potassium 227.9mg 3. Protein

Peanut Butter Oats

Preparation time: 5 mins **Cooking time**: 8 hours **Servings:** 2
Ingredients:
- ½ banana
- ½ c. rolled oats
- 1 tbsp. powdered peanut butter
- ½ c. soymilk
- 1 tbsp. maple syrup
- 1 tbsp. chia seeds
- ½ c. berries
- Salt to taste

Directions:
Take a medium-sized jar and add powdered peanut butter, chia seeds, soymilk, salt, syrup, and oats. Mix everything well. Put the jar in the fridge for a night. Then serve the next day topped with berries or peanut butter.
Nutrition: Calories 368; Fat 9.2g; Carbohydrates 62.8g; Proteins 13.4g; Sodium 239.5mg; Potassium 595.8mg

Breakfast Pizza

Preparation time: 3 mins **Cooking time:** 1 min **Servings:** 2
Ingredients:
- 1 tbsp. pizza sauce
- 1 tbsp. whole wheat bun
- 2 slices provolone cheese
- ½ c. cherry tomatoes

- 1 tbsp. green Pepper
- 1 tbsp. fresh basil
- 1 nectarine

Directions:
Spread pizza sauce on the whole wheat bun. Now place tomatoes, cheese, and peppers on the bun. Cook in the microwave for a minute or until the cheese melts. Garnish with some basil on top and serve along with fresh nectarines on the side.
Nutrition: Calories 295; Fat 8.5g; Carbohydrates 42g; Proteins 17.5g; Cholesterol 21mg; Sodium 502mg.

Breakfast Wraps

Preparation time: 10 mins **Cooking time:** 20 mins **Servings:** 2
Ingredients:
- 2 wheat tortillas
- 3 egg whites
- 1 red pepper
- 1 red onion
- 1 jalapeno pepper
- ½ c. mushrooms
- 1 green pepper
- ¼ c. Mexican cheese blend
- 2 oz. green chilies
- 1 garlic clove
- 1 tsp. olive oil

Directions:
Take a pan and put it on medium-high flame. Heat oil in it. Put garlic, mushrooms, chili, peppers, and onion in the pan and stir-fry them. Take off the pan from heat. Add egg whites with cheese to a bowl and whisk it well. Put another pan on the stove and cook the eggs in it. Make sure eggs are cooked evenly. Now add the egg mixture to the center of the tortilla with the vegetables. Do the same with another tortilla. Then fold the tortilla down to the upper side like a covering on the filling. Place on plates and serve.
Nutrition: Calories 245; Fat 8g; Carbohydrates 29g; Proteins 14g; Cholesterol 5mg; Sodium 446mg; Fiber 4g

Portobello Mushrooms Florentine

Preparation time: 5 mins **Cooking time:** 20 mins **Servings:** 4
Ingredients:
- 4 Portobello mushrooms
- 2 eggs
- ½ c. feta cheese
- 2 c. baby spinach
- 1/8 tsp. garlic salt
- ½ tsp. pepper
- 1 tsp. olive oil
- 2 onions
- 1/8 tsp. salt
- Fresh basil
- Cooking spray

Directions:
Preheat the oven to 425 ° Fahrenheit. Take a baking pan and grease it with cooking spray. Place the mushrooms in the pan and add garlic, salt, and Pepper. Place the pan in the oven for ten minutes, till the mushrooms turn soft. At the same time, the mushrooms are getting tender. Heat some oil in a pan. Put onions in the pan and sauté them till they become soft. Now add spinach to it and let it simmer for a while. Take a bowl and crack the eggs in it, whisk them and add salt. Add the egg mixture to the pan and let them cook with the spinach, stirring in between. When the mushrooms are done, take them out of the oven. When the eggs are cooked, place them over the mushrooms with cheese. Garnish with basil and serve.
Nutrition: Calories 126; Fat 5g; Carbohydrates 10g; Proteins 11g; Cholesterol 18mg; Sodium 472mg; Fiber 3g.

Peanut Butter Oatmeal

Preparation time: 5 mins **Cooking time:** 2 mins **Servings:** 2
Ingredients:
- 2 bananas
- 1 c. oats
- 1 tsp. vanilla extract

- 2 tbsp. peanut butter
- 2 c. milk
- ¼ tsp. salt

Directions:
Pour the milk into a pan and bring it to a boil. Add the oats to it. Let it cook for two minutes but stir in between. Take it off the heat when done, and add the vanilla extract, peanut butter, and salt. Put bananas on top and serve.
Nutrition: Calories 284; Fat 7g; Carbohydrates 47g; Proteins 13g; Cholesterol 4mg; Sodium 260mg; Fiber 5g

Chia Seed Parfaits

Preparation time: 5 mins **Cooking time:** 10 mins **Servings:** 2
Ingredients:
- 1 c. raspberries
- ½ c. blueberries
- ½ c. agave nectar
- 2 tbsp. lemon juice
- 2 tbsp. chia seeds
- 1 tsp. vanilla extract
- 2 tsp. lemon zest
- 1 c. Greek yogurt

Directions:
Take the parfait glasses and add chia seeds, agave nectar, lemon juice, lemon zest, vanilla extract, and Greek yogurt. Make a layer of berries on top. Then repeat the process and make another layer. Serve chilled.
Nutrition: Calories 214; Fat 4g; Carbohydrates 33g; Proteins 13g; Cholesterol 7mg; Sodium 48mg; Fiber 5g.

Breakfast Tacos

Preparation time: 5 minutes **Cooking time:** 15 minutes **Serves** 4
Ingredients:
- 1 avocado, sliced
- 8 egg whites
- 4 corn tortillas
- 1 tablespoon olive oil
- 4 cuts of low-fat turkey bacon, cooked
- ¼ cup chopped tomato

Direction:
Heat olive oil in a medium, nonstick skillet over medium-high heat. Add egg whites and cook until set, about 2 minutes. Warm tortillas according to package directions. Place one tortilla on each of the four plates. Top tortillas with eggs, bacon, tomato, and avocado, and serve.
Nutrition: calories: 210 | fat: 13.5 g | cholesterol: 15 mg|sodium: 343.2 mg| carbohydrates: 8.3 g| fiber: 3.5 g | protein: 13.9 g

Spring Vegetable Frittata

Preparation time: 5 minutes **Cooking time:** 15 minutes **Serves** 2
Ingredients:
- 4 egg whites
- 4 cooked asparagus spears, chopped
- 1 handful of baby spinach leaves
- 1 teaspoon skim milk
- 1 tablespoon olive oil
- ¼ red bell pepper, chopped
- Freshly ground Pepper
- 1-ounce crumbled goat cheese

Direction:
Preheat the broiler. In a small bowl, beat the egg whites with the skim milk until combined. Heat a small, nonstick, ovenproof skillet over medium-high heat. Add the olive oil, followed by the eggs. Spread the spinach on top of the egg mixture in an even layer, and top with the asparagus and red Pepper. Reduce heat to medium, and season with freshly ground Pepper to taste. Cook the eggs and vegetables for 3 minutes, or until the bottom half of the eggs is firm and the vegetables are tender. Top with the crumbled goat cheese, and transfer the skillet to the middle rack under the broiler. Cook another 3 minutes until the eggs are firm in the middle and the cheese has melted. Slice into wedges and serve immediately.
Nutrition: calories: 162.7 | fat: 9.9 g | cholesterol: 6.8 mg|sodium: 215.5 mg| carbohydrates: 4 g| fiber: 1.1 g | protein: 14.7 g

Quiche with Asparagus, Salmon, and Tomato

Preparation time: 10 minutes **Cooking time:** 30 minutes **Serves**: 8
Ingredients:
- 4 ounces smoked salmon, chopped
- 6 asparagus spears, chopped into ½-inch pieces
- 8 egg whites
- 1 tablespoon olive oil
- 1 cup chopped onion
- ½ cup shredded low-fat Cheddar
- ½ cup shredded low-fat mozzarella
- ¼ teaspoon ground white Pepper
- ½ cup halved cherry tomatoes
- Cooking spray

Direction:
Preheat the oven to 350°F. In a medium sauté pan, heat oil over medium-high heat. Add onion and asparagus, and sauté until onion caramelizes for about 8 minutes. Mix egg whites, cheeses, and White Pepper in a large bowl. Gently mix in salmon. Pour the egg mixture into a nonstick pie pan or pan coated with cooking spray. Add tomatoes, placing them in a circle around the outer edge of the egg mixture. Bake for 30 minutes or until eggs is set at the center. Allow resting 5 minutes before serving.
Nutrition: calories: 10 | fat: 4 g | cholesterol: 8.9 mg|sodium: 436 mg| carbohydrates: 4.6 g| fiber: 1.1 g | protein: 4.1 g

Sausage and Egg Sandwich

Preparation time: 10 minutes **Cooking time:** 20 minutes **Serves:** 4
Ingredients:
- 4 egg whites
- 4 slices avocado
- 4 slices tomato
- 1 pound lean ground pork
- 4 whole-grain English muffins, split and toasted
- 4 slices of low-fat Cheddar cheese
- ½ teaspoon ground white Pepper
- 1 teaspoon rubbed sage
- ½ teaspoon dried marjoram
- ½ teaspoon ground ginger
- ⅛ teaspoon ground nutmeg
- Cooking spray

Direction:
Mix well with the pork, white Pepper, sage, marjoram, ginger, and nutmeg in a large bowl. Form into four patties. Heat a nonstick griddle over medium heat. Spray the grill with cooking spray. Add patties to pan, and cook until well-browned and cooked through, about 8 minutes per side. Meanwhile, spray a small, microwave-safe bowl with cooking spray. Add egg whites and microwave on high until cooked (about 2 minutes). Cook an additional 30 seconds if needed. Place the English muffins on a plate and layer the cheese, tomato, avocado, sausage patties, and egg onto the muffins. Serve.
Nutrition: calories: 375 | fat: 12 g | cholesterol: 66 mg|sodium: 532 mg| carbohydrates: 29 g| fiber: 1.2 g | protein: 40.3 g

Tomato Egg Tart

Preparation time: 5 minutes **Cooking Time:** 20 minutes **Serves:** 4
Ingredients:
- 8 large egg whites
- 4 large eggs
- 2 cups artichoke, finely chopped
- ⅓ cup fresh basil, chopped
- 1 cup grape tomatoes, halved
- ¾ tsp freshly ground black Pepper
- ¼ cup low-moisture part-skim ricotta cheese
- Nonstick cooking spray

Directions:
Heat the oven to 400°F gas mark 6. Mix the chopped artichoke, chopped basil, halved tomatoes, ground black pepper, ricotta cheese, large eggs, and egg whites in a large bowl, and combine well. Coat a large oven-safe dish with nonstick cooking spray. Add the mixture to the pan and bake for 20 minutes until the

eggs are cooked, and the edges are slightly browned. Remove from the oven and allow to cool for 10 minutes.
Divide into 4 pieces and serve, or store in the refrigerator for 5 to 7 days.
Nutrition: Calories: 161; Total Fat: 6g; Saturated Fat: 2g; Cholesterol: 169mg; Sodium: 250mg; Total Carbs: 8g; Net Carbs: 2g; Fiber: 4g; Protein: 17g

Spinach Wraps

Preparation Time: 15 Minutes **Cooking time:** 10 minutes **Serves:** 2
Ingredients:
- 3 large eggs
- 2 large whole-grain tortillas
- 1 medium tomato, chopped, divided
- 4 Cheddar cheese slices
- 2 tbsp Tomato Salsa, divided
- 2 cups spinach, divided
- 1 tbsp avocado oil

Directions:
Crack the eggs into a large bowl. Beat gently with a fork. Set out two plates and place a whole-wheat tortilla on each. Place 2 cheddar cheese slices down the middle of each tortilla. Top each with half of the spinach, then half of the tomato and salsa. Heat the avocado oil in nonstick frying over medium heat. Add the beaten eggs and occasionally stir until they are scrambled. Once the eggs are done, spoon them on top of the tomatoes and salsa. Gently fold in the sides of the tortillas and roll them up. Place the wraps, seam-side down, in the pan, cover, and warm through for 2 to 3 minutes over medium heat, watching them not burn. Serve warm.
Nutrition: Calories: 471; Total Fat: 27g; Saturated Fat: 8g; Cholesterol: 300mg; Sodium: 627mg; Total Carbs: 35g; Fiber: 8g; Protein: 22g

Vegetable Shake

Preparation Time: 5 Minutes **Cooking time:** 5 minutes **Serves:** 2
Ingredients:
- 2 cups carrots, chopped
- 2 cups cashew milk
- 2 cups kale, chopped
- 2 tbsp ground flaxseed
- 1 (1½-inch) piece of fresh ginger, peeled
- ½ cup ice

Directions:
Add the chopped carrots, kale, cashew milk, ground flaxseed, and peeled ginger to a blender. Blend for 1 to 2 minutes until smooth, and no lumps remain. Add the ice and blend until smooth. Serve cold.
Nutrition: Calories: 139; Total Fat: 8g; Saturated Fat: 0g; Sodium: 210mg; Total Carbs: 16g; Fiber: 7g; Protein: 5g

Cashew Nut Shake

Preparation Time: 10 Minutes **Cooking time:** 5 minutes **Serves:** 1
Ingredients:
- 2 cups spinach
- ¼ cup unsalted cashew nuts
- 2 tsp unsalted cashew butter
- 1 tbsp unsweetened cacao powder
- ½ medium banana
- 3 oz firm tofu
- 1 cup unsweetened cashew milk

Directions:
Add the spinach, unsweetened cacao powder, cashew butter, banana, firm tofu, milk, and unsalted cashew nuts, and blend on high speed for 1 to 2 minutes until smooth and no lumps remain.
Serve immediately. Tip: for extra flavor, add 1 tsp of vanilla extract in step 1.
Nutrition: Calories: 261; Total Fat: 11g; Saturated Fat: 2g; Cholesterol: 0mg; Sodium: 268mg; Total Carbs: 30g; Net Carbs: 15g; Fiber: 6.5g; Protein: 13g

Hummus and Date Bagel

Preparation time: 3 minutes **Cooking time:** 5 minutes **Serves** 1
Ingredients:
- ¼ serving of Homemade Hummus/store-bought hummus
- 6 dates, pitted &halved
- 1 bagel
- Dash of salt & Pepper to taste
- ¼ cup of diced tomatoes

- 1 tbsp. of chives
- A squeeze of lemon juice
- 1 handful sprouts

Direction:
The bagel is split in half. In a toaster or under the broiler, toast the bagel. Each side is rubbed with hummus. Add the salt, dates, and Pepper to taste.
Nutrition: Calories: 410 kcal, Protein: 91 g, Carbohydrates: 59 g, Fat: 2 g, Cholesterol: 0 mg, Fiber: 9.7 g

Curry Tofu Scramble

Preparation time: 5 minutes **Cooking time:** 5 minutes **Serves** 3
Ingredients:
- 1 teaspoon of curry powder
- 12oz. crumbled tofu
- 1 teaspoon of olive oil
- ¼ cup of skim milk
- ¼ teaspoon of chili flakes

Direction:
In a skillet, heat the olive oil. Toss in the tofu crumbles and chili flakes. Combine skim milk and curry powder in a mixing dish. Stir thoroughly after pouring the liquid over crumbled tofu. On medium-high heat, scramble the tofu for 3 minutes.
Nutrition: Calories: 102 kcal, Protein: 10 g, Carbohydrates: 3.3 g, Fat: 6.4 g, Cholesterol: 0 mg, Fiber: 3 g

Breakfast Splits

Preparation time: 10 minutes **Cooking time:** 0 minutes **Serves** 2
Ingredients:
- 2 peeled bananas
- 4 tablespoons of granola
- 2 chopped strawberries
- 2 tablespoons of low-fat yogurt
- ½ teaspoon of ground cinnamon

Direction:
Combine yogurt, ground cinnamon, and strawberries in a mixing dish. Then cut the bananas lengthwise and fill them with the yogurt mass. Granola may be sprinkled on top of the fruits.
Nutrition: Calories: 154 kcal, Protein: 6.8 g, Carbohydrates: 45.2 g, Fat: 8 g, Cholesterol: 1 mg, Fiber: 4 g

Tomato Basil Bruschetta

Preparation time: 5 minutes **Cooking time:** 0 minutes **Serves** 6
Ingredients:
- 2 tablespoons of chopped basil
- 3 diced tomatoes,
- 1/2 whole-grain baguette, six 1/2-inch-thick diagonal slices
- 1 tablespoon of chopped parsley
- 1/2 cup of diced fennel
- 2 minced cloves of garlic
- 1 teaspoon of olive oil
- 1 teaspoon of black Pepper
- 2 teaspoons of balsamic vinegar

Direction:
Preheat the oven to 400 degrees Fahrenheit. Baguette pieces should be gently toasted. Combine all the remaining ingredients in a large mixing bowl. Distribute the mixture equally over the toasted bread. Serve right away.
Nutrition: Calories: 142 kcal, Protein: 5 g, Carbohydrates: 26 g, Fat: 2 g, Cholesterol: 0 mg, Fiber: 2 g

Creamed Rice

Preparation time: 5 minutes **Cooking time:** 20 minutes **Serves** 2
Ingredients:
- ½ cup brown basmati rice
- 1 cup unsweetened almond milk, plus extra for serving
- 2 cups water
- ⅛ tsp ground cinnamon
- 1 tsp vanilla extract
- ¼ cup dried raisins
- ¼ cup unsalted mixed nuts, chopped

- 2 tbsp. organic honey
- Pinch fine sea salt

Direction:
Place the basmati rice in a large-sized mixing bowl and add the water. Soak overnight in the refrigerator, then drain. Add the soaked rice, water, almond milk, vanilla extract, cinnamon, and fine sea salt to a medium-sized stockpot and place over medium heat. Bring the rice mixture to a boil and reduce the heat to low. Simmer for 20 minutes until the rice is tender and most of the liquid has been absorbed, stirring frequently. Remove the stockpot from the heat and mix in the raisins, nuts, and honey. Add extra almond milk if you prefer a thinner pudding. Serve.
Nutrition: Calories: 340; Total Fat: 8.5g; Saturated Fat: 0g; Cholesterol: 0mg; Sodium: 213mg; Total Carbs: 64g; Net Carbs: 24g; Protein: 6g

Egg Foo Young

Preparation time: 5 minutes **Cooking time:** 10 minutes **Serves** 3
Ingredients:
- 2 ½ cups large egg whites
- ½ medium red bell pepper, chopped
- ½ medium green bell pepper, chopped
- ¼ cup Roma tomatoes, chopped
- ½ tsp basil, chopped
- ¼ cup red onion, finely chopped
- ¼ cup lean ham, chopped
- Cooking spray
- Fine sea salt
- Ground black pepper

Direction:
Spray a medium nonstick frying pan with cooking spray and place it over medium heat. Add the red and green bell peppers, onion, tomato, and ham to the pan and fry for 4 minutes until tender. Add the egg whites into the pan, over the ham mixture, and cook for 1 minute, until just beginning to set. Use a rubber spatula or turner and gently lift the edges of the setting egg whites while tilting the pan to allow any uncooked egg to run beneath. Continue this process for 3 minutes until all the egg whites are set. Remove the pan from the heat and fold one side of the egg white omelet over the other. Cut the omelet in half and sprinkle with chopped basil, seasoned with fine sea salt and ground black Pepper. Serve warm.
Nutrition: Calories: 215; Total Fat: 2g; Saturated Fat: 0g; Cholesterol: 15mg; Sodium: 469mg; Total Carbs: 8g; Net Carbs: 1g; Protein: 40g

Cranberry Hotcakes

Preparation time: 5 minutes **Cooking time:** 9 minutes **Serves** 2
Ingredients:
- 1 large egg
- 1 cup rolled oats
- 1 tbsp. ground flaxseed
- 1 cup cranberries
- 3 tbsp. fat-free plain yogurt
- ¼ cup unsweetened almond milk
- ½ tsp ground cinnamon
- 2 tsp avocado oil

Direction:
Mix the oats, cranberries, yogurt, almond milk, flax seeds, egg, and cinnamon in a medium-sized mixing bowl until it becomes a thick batter. Heat the avocado oil over medium-low heat in a large nonstick frying pan. Pour ¼ cup of the batter into the pan and fry for 2 to 3 minutes, or until bubbles start to form on top, flip, and fry for 2 minutes, or until lightly browned and fully cooked. Continue with the remaining batter. Serve with your favorite toppings.
Nutrition: Calories: 328; Total Fat: 12g; Saturated Fat: 2g; Cholesterol: 83mg; Sodium: 54mg; Total Carbs: 43g; Net Carbs: 10g; Protein: 13g

Chapter 6: Lunch RECIPES

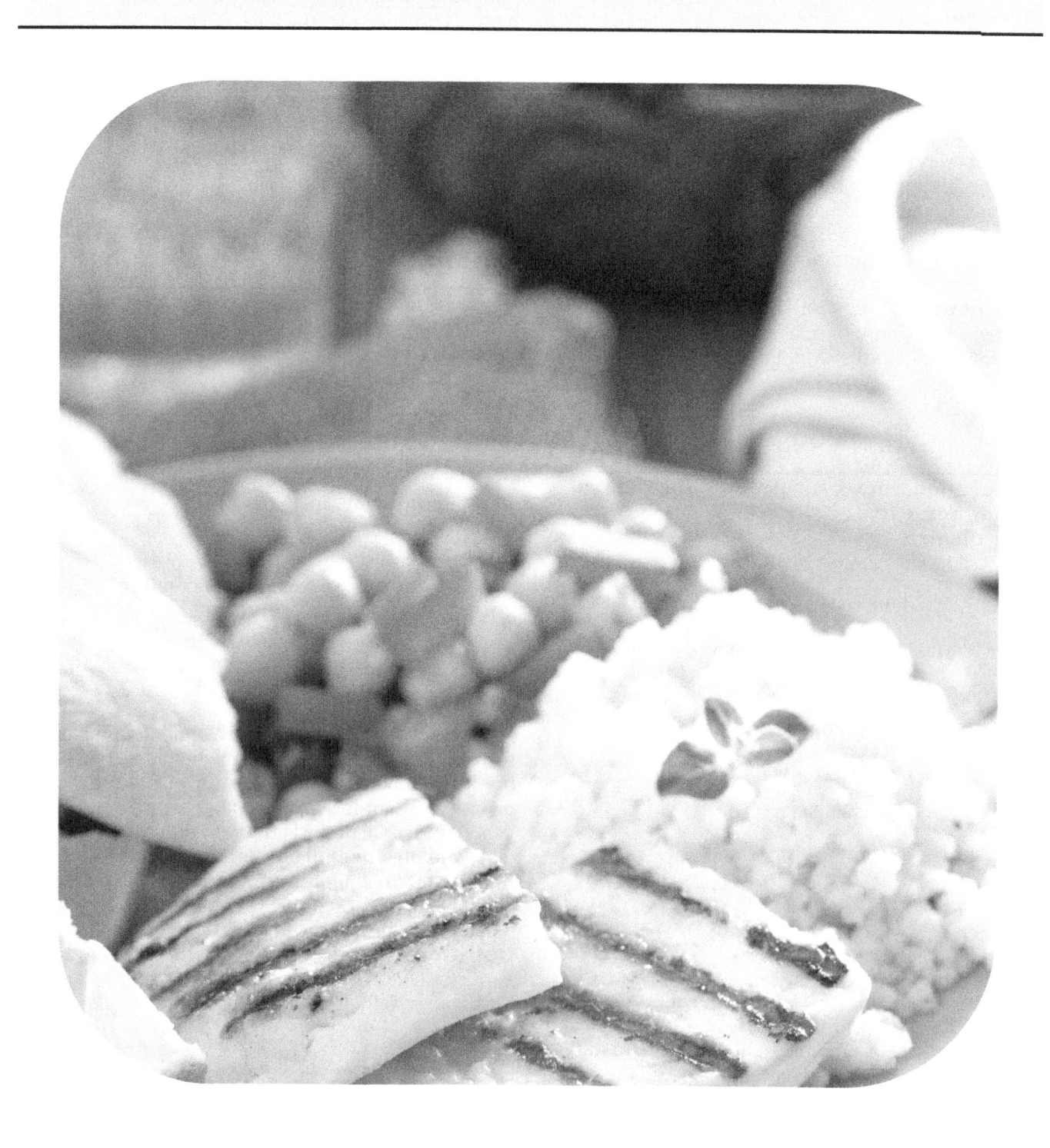

Turkey Keema Curry

Preparation time: 10 minutes **Cooking time:** 40 minutes **Servings:** 4
Ingredients:
- 4 Rotis Coriander
- 2 cup chicken stock
- 2 tsp. ground coriander
- 2 green chilies
- 3 garlic cloves
- 20 oz turkey breast mince
- ½ lemon
- 10 oz frozen peas
- 1 tsp. ground turmeric
- 2 tsp. ground cumin
- Ginger
- 1 onion
- 1 tbsp. vegetable oil
- Tomato Salad Ginger
- 7 oz cherry tomatoes

Directions:
Heat oil in a frying pan. Add the chopped turkey and cook for 5 minutes. Add onions and salt and cook for another 5 minutes. Add chilies, garlic, and ginger and cook for 5 minutes on medium heat. Add spices and stock and simmer for 20 minutes. Add peas, lemon juice, and coriander, and cook for 5 minutes. Mix all the ingredients in a bowl to prepare tomato salad and season. Transfer keema to bowl and serve with salad and rotis.
Nutrition: Calories: 441 kcal | Fat: 9.2 g | Protein: 43.2 g | Carbs: 42.2 g | 32 mg Sodium

Orzo, Bean, and Tuna Salad

Preparation time: 5 minutes **Cooking time:** 10 minutes **Servings:** 2
Ingredients:
- 2 tbsp Chopped dill to taste
- 3 roasted red peppers from a jar
- 1 tbsp. olive oil
- 5 oz green beans
- ½ red onion
- 12 dry-cured black olives
- 1 cup tuna
- 4 oz orzo
- 2 tbsp. sherry vinegar

Directions
Place the onions in a bowl and pour vinegar over it. Boil beans without adding salt for 3 minutes. Remove beans and boil orzo. Rinse and drain. Add dill, peppers, olive oil, beans, olives, tuna, and orzo into the onions bowl. Mix well and serve.
Nutrition: Calories: 298 kcal | Fat: 11.9 g | Protein: 18.7 g | Carbs: 26.6 g | 19 mg Sodium

Smoked Haddock and Spinach Rye Toasts

Preparation time: 10 minutes **Cooking time:** 10 minutes **Servings:** 2
Ingredients:
- 3 long slices of rye bread
- Garlic oil
- ½ cup semi-skimmed milk
- 3 eggs
- 1 oz pecorino Romano
- 7 oz baby spinach
- 7 oz smoked haddock

Directions:
Add water to a pan and boil eggs. Peel and set aside. Place the haddock, milk, and some water in a small pan. Simmer for 3 minutes. Remove the fish and break it into chunks. Add blanched spinach to the bowl and seasoning, ¾ of grated pecorino, and garlic oil. Take the rye toasts and add spinach and haddock over it. Cut the eggs into slices, and add to the toast. Add black pepper and cheese and serve.
Nutrition: Calories: 273 kcal | Fat: 11.1 g | Protein: 29.5 g | Carbs: 12.8 g | 16 mg Sodium

Chipotle Chicken Lunch Wrap

Preparation time: 10 minutes **Cooking time:** 25 minutes **Servings:** 2
Ingredients:
- 4 tbsp Tabasco
- 2 tbsp. soured cream
- 4 tbsp Coriander
- 1 lime
- ¼ red cabbage
- 2 chicken breasts
- 2 tbsp. pickled jalapenos
- 2 large tortilla wraps
- 2 handfuls of baby spinach
- 2 spring onions
- 2 chipotle paste
- 2 chicken breasts

Directions:
Preheat the oven to 350°F. Coat the chicken breasts

with chipotle paste, and season—Bake in the oven for 25 minutes. Add lime juice, spinach, cabbage, coriander, and spring onion to a bowl and mix. Spread sour cream on the tortilla. Add chicken, slaw mix, jalapenos, and Tabasco to the tortilla. Fold the tortilla and cover it in the foil. Slice tortillas in half and serve.
Nutrition: Calories: 329 kcal | Fat: 10 g | Protein: 36.5 g | Carbs: 25.4 g | 20 mg Sodium

Salmon with Marinade

Preparation time: 1 hour 10 mins **Cooking time:** 10 mins **Servings:** 4
Ingredients:
- 1 c. pineapple juice
- 2 garlic cloves
- 2 tsp. soy sauce
- ½ tsp. ginger
- 4 salmon fillets
- ½ tsp. sesame oil
- Black pepper to taste
- 2 c. diced fresh fruit

Directions:
Take a bowl and add ginger, pineapple juice, garlic, and soy sauce. Mix it all well. Take a baking dish and put salmon fillets in it. Drizzle the pineapple mixture on the salmon and let it sit in the fridge for an hour. Set the oven to 375° F. Line a baking tray with aluminum foil squares. Spray the aluminum foil using a cooking spray. Put the salmon in the dish and pour the sesame oil over it. Also, add the fruits on top with black pepper. Cover the salmon with foil entirely and seal the sides, then put the dish in the oven for ten minutes. Once done, dish out and serve immediately.
Nutrition: Calories 247; Fat 7g; Carbohydrates 19g; Proteins 27g; Cholesterol 57mg; Sodium 192mg; Fiber 2g.

Balsamic Roast Chicken

Preparation time: 15 minutes **Cooking time:** 25 minutes **Servings:** 4
Ingredients:
- 1 lb. chicken
- 1 Tbsp. Rosemary
- 2 garlic cloves
- 2 Tbsp. olive oil
- 1/8 tsp. black pepper
- 4 sprigs rosemary
- 1 c. balsamic vinegar
- 1 tsp. brown sugar

Directions:
Set the oven to 350 ° Fahrenheit. In a bowl, mix the garlic with rosemary. Rub the olive oil and the garlic mixture over the chicken flesh. Then add some black pepper and place the rosemary sprigs in the chicken cavity. Put the chicken in a roasting pan and let it roast for twenty-five minutes. When the chicken is roasted, put it on a platter. Take a pan and, put it on heat, add the vinegar with sugar to it. Cook till the sugar dissolves completely. Pour the mixture over the chicken and garnish with rosemary. Then serve immediately.
Nutrition: Calories 301; Fat 13g; Carbohydrates 3g; Proteins 43g; Cholesterol 127mg; Sodium 131mg.

Salad with Balsamic Vinaigrette

Preparation time: 10 minutes **Cooking time:** 5 minutes **Servings:** 4
Ingredients:
- 2 tbsp. balsamic vinegar
- 1/3 c. parsley
- 4 lettuce leaves
- 2 garlic cloves
- ¼ c. olive oil
- 14 oz. garbanzo beans
- 14 oz. black beans
- 1 red onion
- ½ c. celery
- Black pepper to taste

Directions:
Take a bowl and add pepper, parsley, garlic, and vinegar. Whisk everything well. Add olive oil. Keep it aside for now. In another bowl, put the onions with the beans, place the vinaigrette on the mixture, and make sure everything is coated well. Place it in the fridge for a while. Place one lettuce leaf on each plate and add the salad to them. Garnish it with celery. Do the same for other plates, and it's ready to serve.
Nutrition: Calories 206; Fat 10g; Carbohydrates22 g; Proteins 7g; Cholesterol 0mg; Sodium 174mg; Sugar 7g

Beef and Vegetable Kebabs

Preparation time: 10 minutes **Cooking time:** 55 minutes **Servings:** 4
Ingredients:
- ½ c. brown rice
- 2 c. water
- 8 oz. top sirloin
- 2 Tbsp. Italian dressing

- 2 green peppers
- 4 cherry tomatoes
- 2 onions
- 4 wooden skewers

Directions:
Take a pan and put it on high flame. Add some water to the rice and cook till it boils. Then lower the heat and let the rice simmer for forty-five minutes. Then take it out in a bowl. Take a bowl and add the meat, which is cut into pieces in it. Also, drizzle the Italian dressing on top. Mix it well. Cover with a wrapping sheet and put it in the fridge for twenty minutes. Heat the grill and coat it with cooking spray. Set up the cooking rack to a distance of six inches from the heat. Take the skewers and thread the ingredients into them. Two green peppers, two cube meat, two tomatoes, and two onions on each skewer. Place the skewer on the grill and grill them for ten minutes. Turn the sides occasionally so the vegetables and the meat can be cooked evenly. Put the rice on the platter, place the skewer kebab on top, and serve.
Nutrition: Calories 324; Fat 4g; Carbohydrates 54g; Proteins 18g; Cholesterol 39mg; Sodium 142mg; Fiber 4g.

Beef and Vegetable Stew

Preparation time: 5 minutes **Cooking time:** 1-hour **Servings:** 4
Ingredients:
- 1 lb. beef steak
- ½ c. mushrooms
- 2 c. yellow onions
- 1 c. celery
- 1 c. Roma tomatoes
- ½ c. sweet potato
- ½ c. white potato
- 1 c. kale
- 2 tsp. canola oil
- 1 c. carrot
- 4 garlic cloves
- ¼ c. barley
- ¼ c. red wine vinegar
- 2 tsp. balsamic vinegar
- 3 c. vegetable stock
- 1 tsp. sage
- 1 tsp. Thyme -1 tsp. Parsley -1 tsp. oregano
- 1 tsp. Rosemary - Black pepper to taste

Directions:
Heat the broiler on medium flame. Place the steak on it and broil it for fifteen minutes. Don't forget to turn the sides. Once cooked evenly, take them off the heat and keep them aside. Heat oil in a pan over medium flame, then add the vegetables. Stir fry the vegetables for ten minutes. Then put the barley in the pan and cook for another five minutes. Pat dry the steak using paper towels. Put it into the pan with other spices and herbs, vinegar, and stock. Boil it and then let it simmer for another hour. Dish it out when the liquid is thickened, and serve.
Nutrition: Calories 216; Fat 4g; Carbohydrates 24g; Proteins 21g; Cholesterol 46mg; Sodium 138mg; Sugar 7g.

Beef Brisket

Preparation time: 5 mins **Cooking time:** 3 hours **Servings:** 4
Ingredients:
- 2 Tbsp. olive oil
- 1 lb. beef brisket
- Ground pepper to taste
- 1 c. onions
- 2 garlic cloves
- 1 tsp. thyme
- 14 oz. tomatoes
- ½ c. red wine vinegar
- 1 c. beef stock

Directions:
Set the oven to 350 ° Fahrenheit. Take a heavy pot, put it on medium-high heat, and heat some oil. Sprinkle some pepper on the brisket. Cook the meat in portions and ensure it is cooked fully from all sides. Dish out the brisket on a plate. Put the onions in the pot and let them cook till they turn golden. Then add the thyme and garlic and cook for another minute. Now add the tomatoes with broth and vinegar. Let it boil. Then add the beef to the pot and cover it with a lid. Place the pot in the oven and leave it there for two hours to cook. When done, take it out of the range and serve.
Nutrition: Calories 229; Fat 9g; Carbohydrates 6g; Proteins 31g; Cholesterol 95mg; Sodium 184mg.

Caribbean Grilled Pork

Preparation time: 10 minutes **Cooking time:** 10 minutes **Servings:** 2
Ingredients:
- 3 pork loin
- 1 pineapple
- 2 tsp. ginger
- 1 orange
- 2 Tbsp. cilantro
- Juice half a lime

- ½ Tbsp. brown sugar
- 2 tsp. garlic
- 2 tsp. cumin
- 2 tsp. Coriander
- ½ tsp. turmeric
- 2 Tbsp. canola oil

Directions:
Take a bowl and add the fruits with cilantro and lime juice, then place it in the fridge for two days. Mix all the spices and rub them on the pork chops thoroughly. Brush the oil on them. Set up the barbecue and put the chops on the grill. And cook them for five minutes from both sides till they turn brown. Serve them with the refrigerated fruit salsa.
Nutrition: Calories 210; Fat 11g; Carbohydrates 10g; Proteins 19g; Sodium 66mg; Potassium 377mg

Deep, Dark, and Stout Chili

Preparation time: 15 minutes **Cooking time:** 55 minutes **Servings:** 2
Ingredients:
- 2 Tbsp. canola oil
- 1 lb. beef
- 2 c. green bell peppers
- 1 c. red onion
- 2 tomatoes
- 8 oz. kidney beans
- 1 c. dark stout beer
- 2 Tbsp. chili powder
- ½ Tbsp. cumin
- ½ Tbsp. paprika
- 1 Tbsp. beef bouillon granules
- ½ c. cilantro leaves
- ½ c. onion
- 1 lime

Directions:
Cook the beef in a Dutch oven with a bit of oil for four minutes. Put a pan on medium-high flame and heat some oil in it. Add the peppers with onion and sauté them for four minutes. Place the beans, tomatoes, beer, bouillon, paprika, chili, and cumin in the pan and stir. Cook it on low heat for fifty minutes. Once done, take the beef out in a bowl, garnish chilies on top and serve.
Nutrition: Calories 240; Fat 9g; Carbohydrates 19g; Proteins 20g; Sodium 211mg; Potassium 365mg

Grilled Shrimp Tacos

Preparation time: 10 minutes **Cooking time:** 10 minutes **Servings:** 2
Ingredients:
- 6 tortillas
- 1 avocado
- 2 c. lettuce
- 1 Tbsp. lime juice
- ½ c. Pico de Gallo
- 1 clove garlic, chopped
- ¼ tsp. salt
- 1 lb. shrimp
- 2 Tbsp. spices
- ½ c. cilantro leaves

Directions:
Set up the grill and let it heat up. In a bowl, put the avocados and mash them. Then mix the salt, garlic, and lime juice well. Put the shrimps in the mix and coat them well, then take the skewers and add the shrimps to the skewers. Place them on the grill and cook for four minutes. Then take them out from the skewers and put them over the tortillas. Top it up with Pico de Gallo, guacamole, lettuce, and cilantro, and serve.
Nutrition: Calories 286; Fat 10g; Carbohydrates 31g; Proteins 25g; Cholesterol 159mg; Sodium 443mg; Potassium 663mg

Chicken Salad Sandwich

Preparation time: 10 minutes **Cooking time:** 10 minutes **Servings:** 4
Ingredients:
- 2 oz. chicken, boiled and finely chopped
- 1 whole wheat bread
- 2 almonds or cashews
- 1 Tbsp. yogurt
- 1 Tbsp. olive oil
- 1 bunch cilantro
- 4 raisins
- ¼ c. carrot
- ¼ tsp. curry powder
- ⅛ tsp. cumin
- ⅛ tsp. salt
- ⅛ tsp. pepper

Directions:
Take a bowl and then add all the ingredients to it, except the bread slices. Mix them well and make a spread. After toasting the bread, put the spread over them and sprinkle cilantro on top. Cover with another toasted bread slice, then serve.
Nutrition: Calories 326; Fat 20g; Carbohydrates 18g; Proteins 22g; Cholesterol 49mg; Sodium 306mg; Potassium 330mg

Quinoa Bowls with Shrimp

Preparation time: 20 minutes, 4 days **Cooking time:** 10 minutes **Servings:** 2
Ingredients:
- 4 oz. arugula
- 6 oz. shrimp
- ½ c. salad
- 6 oz. quinoa
- ½ c. cheese

Directions:
Start by cooking the quinoa according to the directions mentioned in the pack. Take a bowl and mix the arugula with quinoa and feta. Place it in the fridge for four days. Then take the shrimp, pour cold water over them, and place them in the bowl. Drizzle the salad dressing in the bowl and serve.
Nutrition: Calories 234; Fat 2g; Carbohydrates 29g; Proteins 15g; Cholesterol 53mg; Sodium 184mg; Potassium 379mg

Tomato with Garlicky Chives

Preparation time: 10 minutes **Cooking time:** 20 minutes **Serves** 4
Ingredients:
- 2 pounds of tomatoes, cut into chunks
- 1 bell pepper, cut into chunks
- 1 cucumber, cut into chunks
- 1 small red onion, cut into chunks
- 1 garlic clove, smashed
- 2 teaspoons sherry vinegar
- ½ teaspoon kosher salt
- ¼ teaspoon freshly ground black pepper
- ⅓ cup extra-virgin olive oil Lemon juice (optional)
- ¼ cup fresh chives, chopped, for garnish

Direction:
In a high-speed blender or Vitamix, add the tomatoes, bell pepper, cucumber, onion, garlic, vinegar, salt, and black pepper.
Blend until smooth. With the motor running, add the olive oil and purée until smooth. Add more vinegar or a spritz of lemon juice if needed. Garnish with the chives.
Nutrition: Calories: 240 | Fat:19g | Protein: 4g | Carbohydrates: 18g| Fiber: 5g | Sugar: 11g| Sodium: 155mg

Peppered Cheese with Stocky Cauliflower Soup

Preparation time: 10 minutes **Cooking time:** 25 minutes **Serves** 5
Ingredient:
- 2 tablespoons extra-virgin olive oil
- 1 large head cauliflower, stemmed and chopped
- 3 garlic cloves, minced
- 2 tablespoons dried thyme
- 1 medium onion, diced
- 2½ cups unsalted chicken stock
- ½ teaspoon salt
- 1 teaspoon freshly ground black pepper
- 2 tablespoons unsalted butter
- 2 tablespoons whole wheat flour 2
- ½ cup 1% milk
- ¼ cup grated Parmesan cheese

Direction:
Heat the oil in a large pot over medium-high heat. Sauté the cauliflower, garlic, thyme, and onion for about 2 minutes, stirring frequently. Add the chicken stock, salt, and pepper to taste. Bring to a boil, then reduce to low heat and cook for 20 minutes, or until the vegetables are soft. Meanwhile, melt the butter in a medium saucepan over medium heat. Whisk in the flour for 2 minutes or until well combined. Continue to whisk while gradually adding the milk. Bring to a light boil, stirring constantly, and then remove from the heat. Whisk in the Parmesan cheese once more. Stir in the Parmesan cream sauce until combined with the cauliflower and broth. Allow cooling before dividing the soup into 5 storage containers.
Nutrition: Calories: 240 | Fat: 13g | Protein: 12g | Carbohydrates: 21g| Fiber: 4.5g | Sugar: 4g| Sodium: 446mg

Parsley Chickpea Bowls with Lemon

Preparation time: 10 minutes **Cooking time:** 15 minutes **Serves** 3
Ingredients:
- ⅓ cup tahini
- Juice of 2 large lemons
- 1 teaspoon honey
- 3 tablespoons extra-virgin olive oil, divided
- 2 tablespoons water, plus
- 1¼ cups 2 (15-ounce) cans of no-salt-added chickpeas, drained and rinsed
- ½ teaspoon ground cumin

- ½ teaspoon freshly ground black pepper
- 1 cup whole wheat couscous
- ¼ cup finely chopped fresh parsley
- 2 small cucumbers, peeled and chopped
- 1-pint cherry tomatoes halved
- 1 large green bell pepper, chopped
- 1 medium onion, chopped

Direction:
Whisk together the tahini, lemon juice, honey, and 1 tablespoon of oil in a small bowl. Whisk in 2 tablespoons of water until the mixture is creamy. Set aside. In a medium bowl, stir together the chickpeas, 1 tablespoon of oil, the cumin, and black pepper. Bring the remaining 1¼ cups of water to a boil in a medium saucepan. Add the couscous and return to a spot. Remove from the heat and let rest for 5 minutes. Fluff with the remaining 1 tablespoon of oil and the parsley. In a large bowl, combine the cucumbers, tomatoes, bell pepper, onion, couscous, and chickpea. Add the tahini sauce and mix well. Divide among 4 storage containers.
Nutrition: Calories: 655 | Fat: 24g | Protein: 24g | Carbohydrates: 87g| Fiber: 18g | Sugar: 9g| Sodium: 73mg

Tomato with Cheesy Eggplant Sandwiches

Preparation time: 10 minutes **Cooking time:** 30 minutes **Serves** 2
Ingredients:
- Nonstick cooking spray (optional)
- 1 small eggplant, cut crosswise into ⅓-inch-thick slices
- 1 tablespoon extra-virgin olive oil
- ¼ teaspoon freshly ground black pepper
- 1 tomato, sliced
- 1 small red onion, sliced
- ½ cup chopped fresh basil
- 4 ounces fresh burrata cheese
- 4 whole wheat bread slices

Direction:
Preheat the oven to 375°F. Line a sheet pan with aluminum foil or coat it with nonstick cooking spray. Brush both sides of the eggplant with the oil, put it on the prepared sheet pan, and season with pepper. Roast for about 25 minutes until the skin is wrinkly and the eggplant is soft, and let cool. Divide the roasted eggplant into 2 portions and place in one partition of 2 divided storage containers. Divide the tomato, onion, and basil into the second partition. Store the burrata cheese and bread in their own separate containers. To serve, reheat the eggplant in the microwave for 30 to 1 minute. For each sandwich, toast 2 bread slices. Layer one-quarter of the cheese on a slice of toast and top with the eggplant, tomato, and onion. Add the basil and close the sandwich.
Nutrition: Calories: 542 | Fat: 24g | Protein: 21g | Carbohydrates: 56g| Fiber: 9g | Sugar: 11g| Sodium: 308mg

Lemony Salmon with Spicy Asparagus

Preparation time: 5 minutes **Cooking time:** 20 minutes **Serves** 4
Ingredients:
- 4 (5-ounce) salmon fillets
- 1-pound fresh asparagus ends trimmed, divided
- 2 teaspoons dried dill, divided
- Freshly squeezed lemon juice
- Freshly ground black pepper (optional)
- Lemon wedges for serving

Direction:
Preheat the oven to 450°F. Prepare four 12-by-18-inch sheets of aluminum foil. Spray the center of each sheet of foil with nonstick cooking spray. Place one salmon fillet in the center of each sheet, top with a quarter of the asparagus, ½ teaspoon of dill, and a squeeze of lemon juice. Sprinkle with black pepper (if using). Bring up the sides of the foil and fold the top over twice. Seal the ends, leaving room for air to circulate inside the packet. Repeat with the remaining fillets. Place the packets on a baking sheet and bake for 15 to 18 minutes or until the salmon is opaque. Use caution when opening the packets, as the steam is very hot. Serve with lemon wedges on the side.
Nutrition: Calories: 202 | Fat: 7g | Protein: 31g | Carbohydrates: 5g| Fiber: 3g | Sugar: 0g| Sodium: 110mg

Halibut with Lime and Ginger

Preparation time: 10 minutes **Cooking time:** 10 minutes **Serves** 4
Ingredients:
- 4 (4-ounce) halibut fillets, rinsed and patted dry
- ½ teaspoon freshly ground black pepper
- 3 teaspoons olive oil, divided
- 4 cups of baby spinach
- 1 tablespoon minced peeled ginger
- 2 garlic cloves, minced

- 1 tablespoon balsamic vinegar
- 1 tablespoon freshly squeezed lime juice

Direction:
Sprinkle the fish with black pepper. Using your fingertips, gently press the seasoning to adhere to the fish. In a large nonstick skillet, heat 2 teaspoons of the olive oil over medium-high heat, swirling to coat the bottom. Cook the fish for 2 minutes, or until browned on the bottom. Turn over, and cook for 2 minutes more, or until the fish flakes easily when tested with a fork. Transfer to a plate and cover to keep warm. Heat the remaining 1 teaspoon of olive oil in the same skillet, swirling the bottom to coat. Add the spinach, ginger, and garlic, and cook, constantly stirring, for 2 minutes or until the spinach begins to wilt. Remove the skillet from the heat. Add the balsamic vinegar and lime juice to the spinach and stir. Divide the spinach among four plates and top each serving with a halibut fillet. Serve immediately.
Nutrition: Calories: 162 | Fat: 6g | Protein: 24g | Carbohydrates: 3g| Fiber: 1g | Sugar: 0g| Sodium: 84mg

Lentils & Rice

Preparation time: 20 minutes **Cooking Time:** 40 Minutes **Serves:** 6
Ingredients:
- 6 cups water
- 1 tsp Himalayan pink salt, divided
- 1 cup wild rice
- 1 cup dried brown lentils, picked over
- 3 tbsp olive oil, more if needed
- 2 medium-sized yellow onions, thinly sliced
- ½ cup cilantro, finely chopped
- 6 spring onions, sliced, divided
- Ground black pepper

Directions:
In a large stockpot, bring the water and ¾ tsp of Himalayan pink salt to a boil over high heat. Add the wild rice and cook for 10 minutes. Add the picked-over lentils, and mix to combine. Cover the pot, and simmer for 20 to 25 minutes, or until the lentils and rice are tender. Remove from the heat and drain any remaining liquid. Allow resting for 10 minutes. Heat the olive oil in a large, heavy bottom pan over high heat. Line a plate with paper towels. Add the sliced onions and cook for 20 minutes until well browned. Transfer the onions to the plate to drain. Sprinkle with the remaining ¼ tsp Himalayan pink salt. Mix half the fried onions, the chopped cilantro, and half the sliced spring onion into the lentils and rice mixture. Divide the lentils and rice mixture, and garnish each serving with fried and sliced spring onions. Season with ground black pepper to taste.
Nutrition:: Calories: 333; Total Fat: 10g; Saturated Fat: 7g; Sodium: 399mg; Total Carbs: 50g; Fiber: 6g; Protein: 11g

Cannellini Bean Pizza

Preparation time: 15 minutes **Cooking time:** 15 minutes **Serves:** 3
Ingredients:
- Aluminum foil
- 1½ cups canned cannellini beans drained and rinsed
- ½ cup whole-wheat flour
- 2 large whole eggs
- 1 tbsp nutritional yeast
- 4 tbsp low-sodium tomato puree
- ½ cup entire white mushrooms, thinly sliced
- ½ cup reduced fat cheese blend, shredded
- 1 tbsp garlic, minced
- 1 tsp garlic powder

Directions:
Warm the oven to 450°F, gas mark 8. Line a baking sheet with aluminum foil. Combine the cannellini beans, whole-wheat flour, whole eggs, and nutritional yeast in a food processor or blender. Process for 1 minute until it forms a doughy consistency. Place the bean mixture on the baking sheet, and spread evenly. The combination will not be like pizza dough but slightly sticky. Use a spatula to spread evenly. Bake for 10 minutes, until the edges are lightly browned. Remove the base from the oven, and spread the tomato puree, sliced mushrooms, cheese blend, minced garlic, and garlic powder evenly over the pizza. Bake for 5 minutes, until the cheese, has melted. Cut into 8 slices, and serve warm.
Nutrition: Calories: 291, Total Fat: 9g, Saturated Fat: 3g, Cholesterol: 21mg, Sodium: 206mg, Total Carbs: 36g, Net Carbs: 2.8g, Fiber: 8g, Protein: 19g

Garbanzo Bean Curry

Preparation time: 10 minutes **Cooking time:** 30 minutes **Serves** 4
Ingredients:
- 1 tbsp olive oil
- 1 small onion, finely chopped
- 2 cups stir-fry vegetables, fresh or frozen
- 1 tbsp ginger, grated
- 2 tsp mild curry paste
- 1 tsp ground turmeric
- 1 (14 oz) can dice no-salt-added tomatoes with their juices

- 1 (15 oz) can of garbanzo beans, rinsed and drained
- ¼ cup almond butter
- 2 cups reduced-sodium vegetable stock

Directions:
Heat the olive oil over medium-high heat in a large, heavy-bottom pan. Add the chopped onion, and cook for 4 to 5 minutes, until translucent. Add the stir-fry vegetables, and cook for 3 to 4 minutes. Add the grated ginger, mild curry paste, and ground turmeric, cook for 1 minute, and mix to combine. Stir in the diced tomatoes with their juice, garbanzo beans, almond butter, and vegetable stock, and allow to boil. Allow simmering on low, occasionally stirring, for 5 to 10 minutes, until warmed. Serve hot.
Nutrition: Calories: 308; Total Fat: 14g; Saturated Fat: 1g; Cholesterol: 0mg; Sodium: 348mg; Total Carbs: 34g; Fiber: 10g; Protein: 12g

Potato Salad

Preparation time: 10 minutes **Cooking time:** 0 minutes **Serves** 8
Ingredients:
- 2 tablespoons of minced fresh dill (or 1/2 tablespoon dried)
- 1-pound potatoes, boiled and diced or steamed
- 2 ribs celery, diced (1/2 cup)
- 1 large chopped yellow onion (1 cup)
- 1/4 cup of low-calorie mayonnaise
- 1 large, diced carrot (1/2 cup)
- 1 teaspoon of ground black pepper
- 2 tablespoons of red wine vinegar
- 1 tablespoon of Dijon mustard

Direction:
In a mixing bowl, combine all ingredients and thoroughly mix them. Before serving, chill it.
Nutrition: Calories: 77 kcal, Protein: 1 g, Carbohydrates: 2 g, Fat: 1 g, Cholesterol: 2 mg, Fiber: 1.9 g

Spinach Berry Salad

Preparation time: 10 minutes **Cooking time:** 0 minutes **Serves** 4
Ingredients:
- 1 cup of fresh sliced strawberries
- 4 packed cups of torn fresh spinach
- 1 cup frozen or fresh blueberries
- 1/4 cup of pecan: chopped, toasted.
- 1 small sliced sweet onion,

Salad dressing:
- 2 tablespoons of balsamic vinegar
- 1/8 teaspoon of pepper
- 2 tablespoons of honey
- 2 tablespoons of white wine vinegar or cider vinegar
- 1 teaspoon of curry powder (can be omitted)
- 2 teaspoons of Dijon mustard

Direction:
Toss onion, spinach, blueberries, strawberries, and pecans in a large salad bowl. Combine dressing ingredients in a jar with a tight-fitting cover. Shake it vigorously. Mix the salad in the dressing to coat it. Serve immediately.
Nutrition: Calories: 158 kcal, Protein: 4 g, Carbohydrates: 25 g, Fat: 5 g, Cholesterol: 0 mg, Fiber: 2.3 g

Healthy Minestrone

Preparation time: 12 minutes **Cooking time:** 18 minutes **Serves** 4
Ingredients:
- 1 tablespoon olive oil
- 1 onion, chopped
- 2 cloves garlic, minced
- 1 red bell pepper, seeded and chopped
- 1 cup chopped red cabbage
- 1 (15-ounce can) of low-sodium cannellini beans, rinsed and drained
- 1 (14-ounce) can of no-salt-added diced tomatoes, undrained
- 3 cups low-sodium vegetable broth
- 1 teaspoon dried basil leaves
- ½ teaspoon dried oregano leaves
- ½ teaspoon dried thyme leaves
- Pinch salt
- ⅛ teaspoon black pepper
- ½ cup whole-wheat elbow macaroni
- 2 cups baby spinach leaves
- ¼ cup shredded Parmesan

Direction:
In a large saucepan, heat the olive oil over medium heat. Add the onion and garlic, and cook and stir for 3 minutes. Add the red bell pepper and cabbage, and cook and stir for 2 minutes. Add the beans, tomatoes, broth, basil, oregano, thyme, salt, and pepper. Simmer for 3 minutes. Stir in the macaroni and simmer for 7 to 9 minutes more, or until the pasta is cooked al dente. Stir in the spinach leaves until they wilt, about 1 minute. Serve, topped with the Parmesan cheese.
Nutrition: Calories 290; Fat 6g (with 18% calories

from fat); Saturated fat 1g; Monounsaturated fat 3g; Carbs 45g; Sodium 188mg; Sugar 7g

Quinoa Vegetable Soup

Preparation time: 10 minutes **Cooking time:** 20 minutes **Serves** 4
Ingredients:
- 2 teaspoons olive oil
- 1 leek, white and light-green parts, chopped and rinsed
- 3 cloves garlic, minced
- 2 carrots, sliced ½-inch thick
- 3 cups low-sodium vegetable broth
- 2 tomatoes, chopped
- ¾ cup quinoa, rinsed and drained
- 1 sprig of fresh rosemary
- 1 sprig of fresh thyme
- Pinch salt
- ⅛ teaspoon cayenne pepper
- 1 cup baby spinach leaves

Direction:
In a large saucepan, heat the olive oil over medium heat. Add the leek and garlic, and cook and stir for 2 minutes. Add the carrot, broth, tomatoes, quinoa, rosemary, thyme, salt, and cayenne pepper, and bring to a simmer. Reduce the heat to low, partially cover the pan, and simmer for 17 to 19 minutes, or until the vegetables and quinoa are tender. Stir in the spinach. Remove the rosemary and thyme sprigs, and serve.
Nutrition: Calories 191; Fat 6g (with 28% calories from fat); Saturated fat 1g; Monounsaturated fat 2g; Carbs 32g; Sodium 142mg; Protein 6g; Cholesterol 0mg; Sugar 6g

German Potato Soup

Preparation time: 10 minutes **Cooking time:** 20 minutes **Serves** 4
Ingredients:
- 2 teaspoons olive oil
- 2 onions, chopped
- 4 cloves garlic, minced
- 2 large Yukon Gold potatoes, rinsed and chopped
- 2 cups low-sodium vegetable broth
- 1 tablespoon low-sodium yellow mustard
- 1 teaspoon tamari sauce
- 1 tablespoon chopped fresh rosemary leaves
- ½ teaspoon dried sage leaves
- ¼ cup plain low-fat Greek yogurt
- ¼ cup grated extra sharp cheddar cheese
- ⅓ cup chopped fresh flat-leaf parsley
- ¼ cup vegan bacon bits (optional)

Direction:
In a large saucepan, heat the olive oil over medium heat. Add the onions and garlic, and cook and stir for 3 minutes. Add the potatoes, vegetable broth, mustard, tamari, rosemary, and sage to a simmer. Simmer for 14 to 17 minutes or until the potatoes are tender. At this point, some of the soup needs to be puréed, and there are many methods you can choose from. You can do this with an immersion blender, leaving some potato chunks whole if you'd like. You can use a potato masher right in the pot. Or put half of the soup into a blender, cover the blender with the lid and a towel, and blend until smooth. Then pour the blended mixture back into the soup. After you have puréed the soup, stir in the yogurt and cheddar cheese. Simmer the soup for 1 minute, then ladle it into bowls. Garnish with parsley and vegan bacon bits if using.
Nutrition: Calories 223; Fat 5g (with 20% calories from fat); Saturated fat 2g; Carbs 37g; Sodium 208mg; Protein 8g; Cholesterol 8mg;

Pasta Primavera

Preparation time: 10 minutes **Cooking time:** 30 minutes **Serves** 6
Ingredients:
- 1 cup of sliced yellow squash or zucchini
- 1 cup of sliced mushrooms
- 2 cups of broccoli florets
- 1 tablespoon of olive oil; extra-virgin
- 2 cups of shredded green or red peppers
- 2 minced garlic cloves,
- 1/2 cup of chopped onion
- 1 cup of evaporated fat-free milk
- 1 teaspoon of butter
- 3/4 cup of Parmesan cheese; freshly grated.
- 1/3 cup of fresh, finely chopped parsley.
- 12 ounces of whole-wheat pasta

Direction:
Bring 1 inch of water to a boil in a big saucepan with a steamer basket. Add mushrooms, zucchini, broccoli, and peppers. Cover and steam for 10 minutes, or until tender-crisp. Remove the saucepan from the heat. Heat the olive oil in a wide saucepan and sauté the garlic and onion over medium heat. Stir or shake the steamed veggies to cover them evenly in the garlic and onion mixture. Remove the pan from the heat but keep it warm. Heat the milk, butter, and

Parmesan cheese in a separate wide pot. Stir constantly over low heat until the sauce has thickened and cooked thoroughly. Stir constantly to avoid scalding. Remove the pan from the heat but keep it warm. Fill a big saucepan 3/4 full of water and bring to a boil in the meanwhile. Cook pasta for 10 to 12 minutes, or according to package instructions, until the pasta is al dente (tender). Drain all of the water from the pasta. Distribute the spaghetti equally among the plates. Pour the sauce over the after topping with vegetables. Serve immediately with fresh parsley as a garnish.

Nutrition: Calories: 347 kcal, Protein: 17 g, Carbohydrates: 54 g, Fat: 7 g, Cholesterol: 12 mg, Fiber: 4 g

Chapter 7: DINNER RECIPES

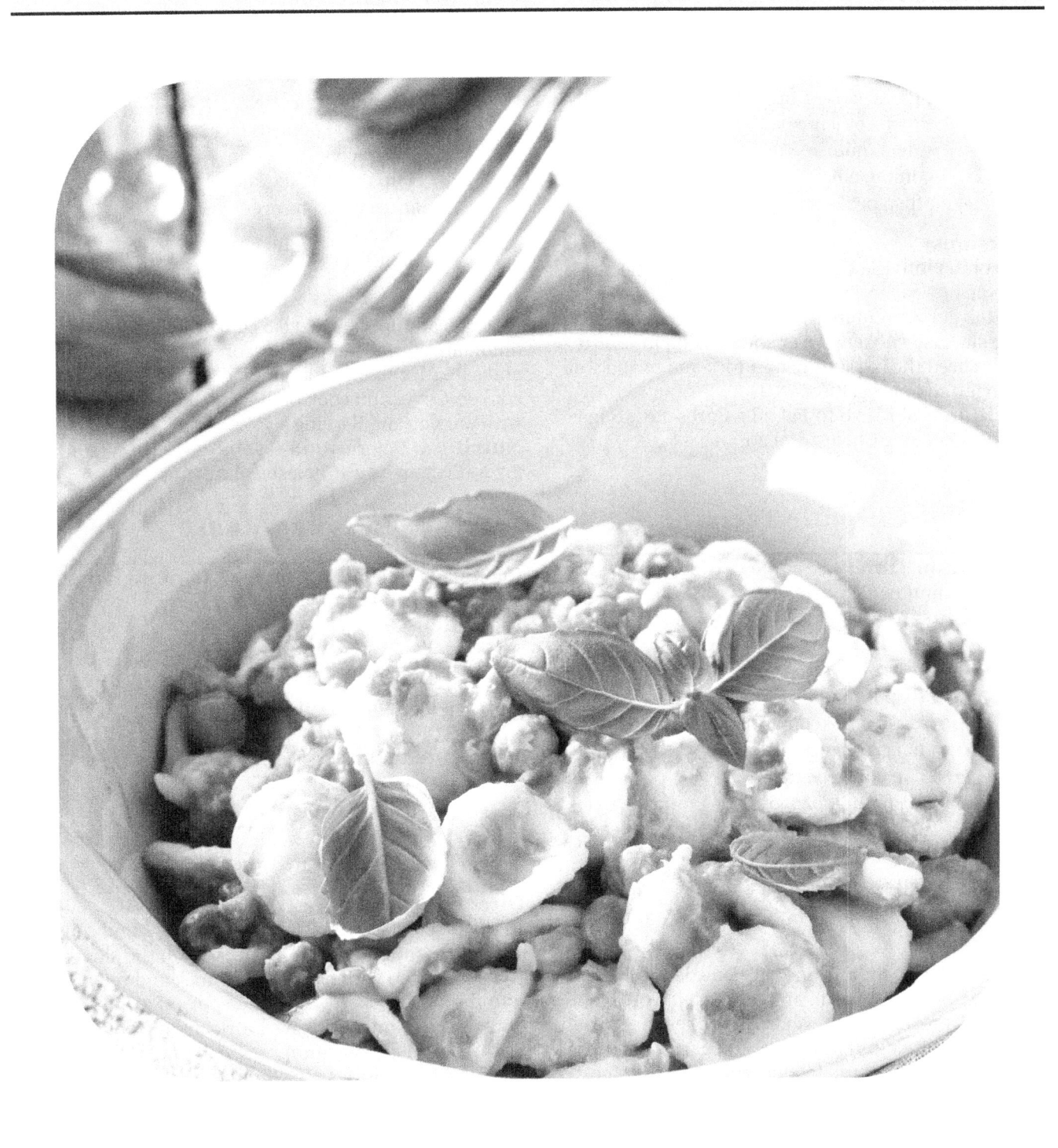

Smoky Hawaiian Pork

Preparation Time: 10 minutes **Cooking Time:** 6 Hours **Servings:** 6
Ingredients:
- 4 lbs. pork cook
- 2 garlic cloves, minced
- 2 tbsp soy sauce
- 4 tbsp fluid smoke
- 1 onion, cut
- 1 tbsp ocean salt

Directions:
Place onion into the sluggish cooker. In a little bowl, combine one garlic, soy sauce, fluid smoke, and ocean salt. Rub garlic combination all over pork. Place pork in the sluggish cooker. Cover and cook on low for 6 hours. Shred the pork utilizing a fork and mixed well. Servings and appreciation.
Nutrition: Calories 640 Fat 28 g Carbs 2.8 g Sugar 0.9 g Protein 47 g Cholesterol 260 mg

Chipotle Tacos

Preparation Time: 10 minutes **Cooking Time:** 8 Hours 10 minutes **Servings:** 10
Ingredients:
- 2 1/2 lbs. meat throw broil
- 1 tbsp olive oil
- 1 tbsp Italian flavoring
- 1/2 tsp smoked paprika
- 1 tsp ground cumin
- 1 cup chicken stock
- 2 tbsp tomato glue
- 1 tbsp chipotle in adobo sauce, minced
- 3 garlic cloves, minced
- 1 tsp stew powder
- 1 tsp salt

Directions:
In a little bowl, combine one stew powder, Italian flavoring, paprika, cumin, and salt. Rub flavors blend, toss meal, and spot in the sluggish cooker. Heat oil in a skillet over medium intensity. Add garlic and sauté for 2 minutes. Add tomato glue, chipotle, and stock and mix well. Remove skillet from heat and pour stock combination over meat. Cover and cook on low for 8 hours. Shred the beef utilizing a fork and Serving.
Nutrition: Calories 438 •Fat 33 g •Starches 1.5 g • Sugar 0.6 g •Protein 30g •Cholesterol 118 mg

Zesty Pepper Beef

Preparation Time: 10 minutes **Cooking Time:** 4 Hours **Servings:** 6
Ingredients:
- 2 lbs. hamburger toss, cut
- 1 cup chicken stock
- 1 little onion, cut
- 2 cups chime pepper, cleaved
- 1 tsp sriracha sauce
- 1/3 cup parsley, hacked
- 2 garlic cloves, minced
- 1 tsp pepper
- 2 tsp salt

Directions:
Place meat into the sluggish cooker and top with onion and chime pepper. Season with garlic, pepper, and salt. Mix stock and sriracha and fill the slow cooker. Cover and cook on high for 4 hours. Garnish with parsley and Serving.
Nutrition: Calories 308 •Fat 9.8 g •Carbs 5 g •Sugar 2.7 g •Protein 47 g •Cholesterol 135 mg

Italian Roast

Preparation Time: 10 minutes **Cooking Time:** 8 Hours **Servings:** 8
Ingredients:
- 2 1/2 lbs. hamburger round broil
- 1/2 cup chicken stock
- 1 little onion, cut
- 1/2 tsp marjoram
- 1/2 tsp thyme
- 1 ½ tsp basil
- 1/2 cup red wine
- 1/4 tsp pepper
- 1 tsp fit salt

Directions:
In a little bowl, combine as one all flavors and rub all over the hamburger cook. Place meal in the sluggish cooker and top with onion. Pour stock and red wine into the slow cooker. Cover and cook on low for 8 hours. Shred meat utilizing a fork and mixed well. Servings and appreciation.
Nutrition: •Calories 284 •Fat 11 g •Sugars 1.4 g • Sugar 0.5 g •Protein 39 g •Cholesterol 122 mg

Yummy Steak Bites

Preparation Time: 10 minutes **Cooking Time:** 8 Hours **Servings:** 4
Ingredients:
- 3 lbs. round steak, cut into 1-inch blocks

- 1/2 cup chicken stock
- 4 tbsp margarine, cut
- 1 tsp garlic powder
- 1 tbsp onion, minced
- 1/2 tsp pepper
- 1/2 tsp salt

Directions:
Place meat shapes into the sluggish cooker and pour stock over the meat. Sprinkle with garlic powder, onion, pepper, and salt. Place margarine cuts on top of the meat. Cover and cook on low for 8 hours. Servings and appreciation.
Nutrition: Calories 845 •Fat 44 g •Starches 1 g • Sugar 0.4 g •Protein 47 g •Cholesterol 320 mg

Teff with Broccoli Pesto

Preparation time: 10 minutes **Cooking time:** 20 minutes **Serving:** 4
Ingredients:
- 3½ cups low-sodium vegetable broth, divided
- 1 cup teff
- 1½ cups broccoli florets, cut into bite-sized pieces
- 1 cup packed fresh basil leaves
- 2 tablespoons fresh lemon juice
- 1/8 teaspoon black pepper
- 2 tablespoons olive oil
- 2 tablespoons grated Romano cheese
- 2 cloves garlic
- Pinch salt

Direction:
Bring 2½ cups of the vegetable broth to a boil in a medium saucepan. Add the teff and bring it back to a simmer. Reduce the heat to low and simmer for 15 to 20 minutes or until the teff is tender. Meanwhile, in another medium saucepan, combine the broccoli and the remaining 1 cup of vegetable broth over medium heat and bring to a simmer. Simmer for 5 to 7 minutes or until the broccoli is tender. Drain, reserving 2 tablespoons of vegetable broth. To make the broccoli pesto, put the broccoli in a food processor or blender and add the basil, olive oil, lemon juice, Romano cheese, garlic, reserved vegetable broth, salt, and pepper. Process or blend until the mixture is smooth.
Drain the teff, if necessary, and place in a serving bowl. Toss half the broccoli pesto with the teff, and drizzle the remaining broccoli mixture. Serve immediately.
Nutrition: Calories 286; Fat 9g (with 28% calories from fat); Saturated fat 2g; Monounsaturated fat 4g; Carbs 41g; Sodium 168mg; Protein 11g; Cholesterol 4mg; Sugar 2g

Warm Barley Salad with Spring Veggies

Preparation time: 10 minutes **Cooking time:** 20 minutes **Serving:** 4
Ingredients:
- 1 cup quick-cooking pearled barley
- 2½ cups low-sodium vegetable broth
- 1 tablespoon olive oil
- ½ pound asparagus spears, cut into 1-inch pieces, tough stem removed
- 4 scallions, chopped
- 1 cup sugar snap peas
- 2 cups frozen baby peas, thawed
- 2 tablespoons fresh lemon juice
- 2 tablespoons low-sodium yellow mustard
- 2 tablespoons apple juice
- 2 teaspoons fresh thyme leaves

Direction:
In a large saucepan, combine the barley and broth over medium-high heat and bring to a boil. Reduce the heat to low, partially cover, and simmer until the barley is tender, 10 to 15 minutes. Meanwhile, heat the olive oil in a large non-stick skillet. Add the asparagus, scallions, and sugar snap peas. Sauté until the vegetables are crisp-tender. Add the baby peas, and cook 1 minute. Mix the lemon juice, mustard, apple juice, and thyme in a large serving bowl. Add the sautéed vegetables to the bowl.
Drain the barley, if necessary, and add to the bowl along with the sautéed vegetables and dressing. Toss to coat, and serve warm.
Nutrition: Calories 357; Fat 5g (with 13% calories from fat); Saturated fat 1g; Monounsaturated fat 2g; Carbs 69g; Sodium 103mg;; Protein 12g; Cholesterol 0mg; Sugar 19g

Roasted Shrimp and Veggies

Preparation time: 10 minutes **Cooking time:** 20 minutes **Serving:** 4
Ingredients:
- 1 cup sliced cremini mushrooms
- 2 medium chopped Yukon Gold potatoes, rinsed, unpeeled
- 2 cups broccoli florets
- 3 cloves garlic, sliced
- 1 cup sliced fresh green beans
- 1 cup cauliflower florets
- 2 tablespoons fresh lemon juice

- 2 tablespoons low-sodium vegetable broth
- 1 teaspoon olive oil
- 1 teaspoon dried thyme
- ½ teaspoon dried oregano
- Pinch salt
- 1/8 teaspoon black pepper
- ½ pound medium shrimp, peeled and deveined

Direction:
Preheat the oven to 400°F. In a large baking pan, combine the mushrooms, potatoes, broccoli, garlic, green beans, and cauliflower, and toss to coat. In a small bowl, mix the lemon juice, broth, olive oil, thyme, oregano, salt, and pepper. Drizzle over the vegetable Roast for 15 minutes, then stir. Add the shrimp and distribute it evenly. Roast for another 5 minutes or until the shrimp curl and turn pink. Serve immediately.
Nutrition: Calories 192; Fat 3g (with 14% calories from fat); Saturated fat 0g; Monounsaturated fat 1g; Carbs 29g; Sodium 116mg; Protein 17g; Cholesterol 86mg; Sugar 3g

Shrimp and Pineapple Lettuce Wraps

Preparation time: 15 minutes **Cooking time:** 12 minutes **Serving:** 4
Ingredients:
- 2 teaspoons olive oil
- 2 jalapeño peppers, seeded and minced
- 6 scallions, chopped
- 2 yellow bell peppers, seeded and chopped
- 8 ounces small shrimp, peeled and deveined
- 2 cups canned pineapple chunks, drained, reserving juice
- 2 tablespoons fresh lime juice
- 1 avocado, peeled and cubed
- 1 large carrot, coarsely grated
- 8 romaine or Boston lettuce leaves, rinsed and dried

Direction:
In a medium saucepan, heat the olive oil over medium heat.
Add the jalapeño pepper and scallions and cook for 2 minutes, stirring constantly. Add the bell pepper, and cook for 2 minutes. Add the shrimp, and cook for 1 minute, stirring constantly.
Add the pineapple, 2 tablespoons of the reserved pineapple juice, and lime juice, and bring to a simmer. Simmer for 1-minute longer or until the shrimp curl and turn pink. Let the mixture cool for 5 minutes. Serve the shrimp mixture with the cubed avocado and grated carrot, wrapped in the lettuce leaves.
Nutrition: Calories 241; Fat 9g (with 33% calories from fat); Saturated fat 2g; Monounsaturated fat 5g; Carbs 29g; Sodium 109mg; Protein 6g; Cholesterol 109mg; Sugar 16g

Grilled Scallops with Gremolata

Preparation time: 15 minutes **Cooking time:** 6 minutes **Serving:** 4
Ingredients:
- 2 scallions, cut into pieces
- ¾ cup packed fresh flat-leaf parsley
- ¼ cup packed fresh basil leaves
- 1 teaspoon lemon zest
- 3 tablespoons fresh lemon juice
- 1 tablespoon olive oil
- 20 sea scallops
- 2 teaspoons butter, melted
- Pinch salt
- 1/8 teaspoon lemon pepper

Direction:
Prepare and preheat the grill to medium-high. Make sure the grill rack is clean. Meanwhile, make the gremolata. In a blender or food processor, combine the scallions, parsley, basil, lemon zest, lemon juice, and olive oil. Blend or process until the herbs are finely chopped. Pour into a small bowl and set aside. Put the scallops on a plate. If the scallops have a small tough muscle attached to them, remove and discard it. Brush the melted butter over the scallops. Sprinkle with salt and lemon pepper. Place the scallops in a grill basket if you have one. If not, place a sheet of heavy-duty foil on the grill, punch some holes in it, and arrange the scallops evenly across it. Grill the scallops for 2 to 3 minutes per side, turning once, until opaque. Drizzle with the gremolata and serve.
Nutrition: Calories 190; Fat 7g (with 33% calories from fat); Saturated fat 2g; Monounsaturated fat 3g; Carbs 2g; Sodium 336mg; Protein 28g; Cholesterol 68mg; Sugar 1g

Healthy Paella

Preparation time: 15 minutes **Cooking time:** 15 minutes **Serving:** 4
Ingredients:
- 1 tablespoon olive oil
- 1 onion, chopped
- 3 cloves garlic, minced
- 1 red bell pepper, seeded and chopped

- 2½ cups low-sodium vegetable broth
- 1 tomato, chopped
- 1 teaspoon smoked paprika
- 1 teaspoon dried thyme leaves
- ¼ teaspoon turmeric
- 1/8 teaspoon black pepper
- 1 cup whole-wheat orzo
- ½ pound halibut fillets, cut into 1-inch pieces
- 12 medium shrimp, peeled and deveined
- ¼ cup chopped fresh flat-leaf parsley

Direction:
In a large deep skillet, heat the olive oil over medium heat. Add the onion, garlic, and red bell pepper, and cook for 2 minutes. Add the vegetable broth, tomato, paprika, thyme, turmeric, and black pepper to a simmer. Stir in the orzo, making sure it is submerged in the liquid in the pan. Simmer for 5 minutes, stirring occasionally. Add the halibut and stir. Simmer for 4 minutes. Add the shrimp and stew. Simmer for 2 to 3 minutes or until the shrimp curl and turn pink and the pasta is cooked al dente. Sprinkle with the parsley, and serve immediately.
Nutrition: Calories 367; Fat 7g (with 17% calories from fat); Saturated fat 1g; Monounsaturated fat 3g; Carbs 50g; Sodium 147mg; Protein 25g; Cholesterol 50mg; Sugar 5g

Baked Pork Chops

Preparation time: 10 minutes **Cooking time:** 20 minutes **Servings:** 6
Ingredients:
- ½ tsp. Salt
- 1/8 tsp. cayenne pepper
- ½ tsp. garlic powder
- 2 tsp. oregano
- ¼ cup fine dry breadcrumbs
- 1 cup evaporated skim milk
- 6 lean center-cut pork chops
- 1/8 tsp. dry mustard
- ½ tsp. black pepper
- ¾ tsp. chili powder
- 4 tsp. paprika
- ¾ cup cornflake crumbs
- 1 egg white

Direction:
Preheat the oven to 375°F. Take pork chops and trim the fat in a bowl mix the egg and milk. Add chops and set aside. In another bowl, mix spices, salt, breadcrumbs, and cornflakes. Drizzle cooking spray in a pan. Remove chops from the milk and coat with crumbs. Transfer them to a baking pan and bake for 20 minutes. Remove the pan from the oven and serve.
Nutrition: Calories: 216 kcal | Fat: 8 g | Protein: 25 g | Carbs: 10 g | 17 mg Sodium

Shish Kabob

Preparation time: 15 minutes **Cooking time:** 15 minutes **Servings:** 8
Ingredients:
- 24 small onions
- 24 cherry tomatoes
- 1/8 tsp. black pepper
- ¼ tsp. salt
- 1 lemon
- ½ cup chicken broth
- 24 mushrooms
- 2 lb. lean lamb
- ½ tsp. rosemary
- 1 tsp. chopped garlic
- ¼ cup red wine
- 2 tbsp. olive oil

Directions
Mix wine, pepper, salt, oil, lemon juice, rosemary, garlic, and broth in a bowl. Dip lamb and mushrooms, tomatoes, and onion in it and put in the fridge for 15 minutes. Take skewers and string lamb, tomatoes, mushrooms, and onions on skewers. Broil for 15 minutes. Serve and enjoy!
Nutrition: Calories: 274 kcal | Fat: 12 g | Protein: 26 g | Carbs: 16 g | 20 mg Sodium

Spicy Veal Roast

Preparation time: 25 minutes **Cooking time:** 1 hour 30 minutes **Servings:** 12
Ingredients:
- 1 bay leaf
- 4 sprigs of fresh parsley
- ½ clove of garlic
- 4 tsp. olive oil
- 1 ½ tsp. cumin
- ½ tsp. black pepper
- 1 tsp. thyme
- 2 tsp. dried tarragon
- ½ lb. onions
- 3 lb. boned lean veal shoulder
- ½ tsp. cinnamon
- ¼ tsp. salt

Direction:
Combine cumin, pepper, cinnamon, and salt and rub

it over the roast. Heat the oil in a pan. Add garlic, onions, and tarragon. Cook for 10 minutes. Take another pan, heat the remaining oil, and add the meat, onion, garlic, and tarragon, along with parsley, bay leaf, and thyme. Place in the oven for one and a half hours at 325°F. Serve and enjoy!
Nutrition: Calories: 206 kcal | Fat: 8 g | Protein: 30 g | Carbs: 2 g | 17 mg Sodium

Barbecued Chicken

Preparation time: 15 minutes **Cooking time:** 60 minutes **Servings:** 8
Ingredients:
- 1 cup chicken broth
- 1 tbsp. hot pepper flakes
- 2 tbsp. brown sugar
- 3 tbsp. vinegar
- 3 lb. chicken parts
- 1 tbsp. chili powder
- Black pepper
- 3 tbsp. Worcestershire sauce
- 1 large onion

Direction:
Add the chicken to a pan and the onions on top. Add Worcestershire sauce, chili powder, pepper, vinegar, stock, hot pepper flakes, and brown sugar. Mix well. Place it in the oven for 1 hour at 350°F. Serve and enjoy!
Nutrition: Calories: 176 kcal | Fat: 6 g | Protein: 24 g | Carbs: 7 g | 11 mg Sodium

Barbecued Chicken-Spicy

Preparation time: 1 hour **Cooking time:** 30 minutes **Servings:** 6 **Difficult**
Ingredients:
- 1 ½ lb. chicken
- 5 tbsp. tomato paste
- 2 cloves garlic
- 1 tsp. ketchup
- ⅛ tsp. black pepper
- 4 tsp. white vinegar
- 1 tsp. molasses
- ⅛ tsp. ginger
- 1 tsp. Worcestershire sauce
- ¼ tsp. onion powder
- ¾ tsp. cayenne pepper
- 2 tsp. honey

Direction:
In a pan, combine all the ingredients except for the chicken. Allow it to simmer for 15 minutes. Take the chicken and brush it with sauce. Marinate the chicken in the fridge for 1 hour. Coat a baking sheet with baking foil. Place chicken in it, add the remaining sauce, and bake for 30 minutes at 350°F. Serve and enjoy!
Nutrition: Calories: 176 kcal | Fat: 4 g | Protein: 27 g | Carbs: 7 g | 9 mg Sodium

Glazed Meatloaf

Preparation time: 25 minutes **Cooking time:** 1 hour **Servings:** 10
Ingredients:
- 1 egg
- ½ cup unsalted ketchup
- 1 tbsp. dry mustard
- 2 tbsp. poultry seasoning
- ½ cup chopped bell pepper
- 2 lbs. hamburger
- 1 tbsp. balsamic vinegar
- ½ cup no salt cracker meal
- 1 tbsp. dry mustard
- 2 tbsp. Kitchen Bouquet
- ½ cup onion

For Glaze
- 1 tbsp. Kitchen Bouquet
- 2 tbsp. dry mustard
- 1 ½ cup no-salt tomato sauce
- 4 tbsp. cider vinegar
- 4 tbsp. brown sugar

Direction:
Combine all the ingredients in a bowl. Shape the mixture into a loaf shape on a baking sheet. Bake for an hour at 350°F. Prepare the glaze by mixing all the ingredients in a different bowl. Pour the glaze over the meat and serve.
Nutrition: Calories: 248 kcal | Fat: 11 g | Protein: 19 g | Carbs: 14 g | 18 mg Sodium

Chicken with Tarragon and Lentils, Pan-Roasted

Preparation time: 15 minutes **Cooking time:** 60 minutes **Servings:** 8
Ingredients:
- 4 shallots
- 4 sweet potatoes
- 1 tbsp. fresh chopped tarragon
- 1 cup dried French green lentils
- 2 tbsp. golden balsamic vinegar
- 1 tbsp. olive oil

- ¼ tsp. poultry seasoning
- 2 cup chicken broth
- 1 cup dry white wine
- 3 garlic cloves
- Fresh ground pepper
- Salt
- 4 lb. whole chicken split down the back

Direction:
Preheat the oven to 350°F. Take potatoes, wrap them in foil, and bake in the oven for 45 minutes. Rinse chicken and remove fat from it. Sprinkle ground pepper and poultry seasoning over it. Heat olive oil in a pan. Add chicken breasts to it—Cook for 10 minutes. Add garlic and shallots and cook for another minute. Add wine, balsamic vinegar, and broth to the pan and stir. Add lentils and ground pepper. Place the pan in the oven at 350°F for 43 minutes. Transfer to a plate and serve with mashed potatoes and lentils.
Nutrition: Calories: 352 kcal | Fat: 8 g | Protein: 36 g | Carbs: 27 g | 20 mg Sodium

Chicken with Lemon Pepper and Garlic

Preparation time: 15 minutes **Cooking time:** 15 minutes **Servings:** 4
Ingredients:
- 1 cup Rice
- 2 tbsp. Lemon pepper and garlic marinade and Sauce
- 1 medium shallot
- 1 ½ cup portabella mushrooms
- Olive oil cooking spray
- Golden balsamic vinegar
- 2 garlic cloves
- 2 boneless chicken breasts

Direction:
Place the chicken in a pan. Coat it with olive oil. Cook chicken over medium heat. Add garlic and shallots and cook for 1 minute. Add mushrooms and golden balsamic vinegar and stir. Add lemon pepper and garlic sauce and simmer on low flame. Serve with boiled Rice and steamed vegetables.
Nutrition: Calories: 256 kcal | Fat: 3 g | Protein: 29 g | Carbs: 26 g | 21 mg Sodium

Teriyaki Chicken with Black Rice and Vegetables

Preparation time: 10 minutes **Cooking time:** 20 minutes **Servings:** 4
Ingredients:
- 2 tbsp. Plus 1 tsp. bottled teriyaki sauce
- 12 oz. package of frozen vegetables
- 2 cups cooked Chinese Black rice
- Asparagus
- 2 boneless chicken breasts
- Baby carrot blend
- White corn

Direction:
Boil rice according to the instructions on the package without adding salt. Place the chicken in a pan. Coat it with olive oil. Cook on medium heat. Add Teriyaki sauce and cook for another minute. Boil frozen vegetables with no salt. Transfer chicken, Rice, and vegetables to the plate and serve.
Nutrition: Calories: 278 kcal | Fat: 3 g | Protein: 26 g | Carbs: 31 g | 22 mg Sodium

Sweet and Sour Chicken with Rice

Preparation time: 20 minutes **Cooking time:** 20 minutes **Servings:** 4
Ingredients:
- 2 boneless chicken breasts
- 1 tbsp. poultry seasoning
- Sliced scallions
- Salt-free seasoning
- ½ cup Sweet and Sour Sauce
- Olive oil
- 1 tbsp. marjoram
- ¼ cup all-purpose flour
- Sesame seeds to taste
- 1 cup uncooked Rice
- ¼ cup water and ¼ cup milk mixed
- 1 tsp. Salt-Free Riley's
- 1 tbsp. granulated garlic
- ¼ cup cornmeal

Direction:
Combine marjoram in a bowl, Riley's All-Purpose seasoning, cornmeal, granulated garlic, flour, and poultry seasoning. Dip the chicken breasts in the milk and water mixture, coat them with the seasoning in a pan, and heat olive oil. Place the chicken in the pan and cook for a few minutes. Boil rice without adding salt. Add Sweet and Sour Sauce to a bowl and microwave to warm it. Pour the sauce over the chicken. Transfer chicken and serve with Rice,

steamed vegetables, and sliced scallions.
Nutrition: Calories: 457 kcal | Fat: 4 g | Protein: 32 g | Carbs: 62 g | 30 mg Sodium

Pasta with Vegetables

Preparation time: 10 minutes **Cooking time:** 40 minutes **Servings:** 2
Ingredients:
- 8 oz. spaghetti
- 2 red peppers, diced
- 1/2 tsp. garlic, chopped
- 2 Tbsp. olive oil
- 1 zucchini, sliced
- 4 tomatoes, cubed
- 1 tsp. sugar
- 2 Tbsp. onion, chopped
- 1 Tbsp. basil
- ½ tsp. oregano
- 1/8 tsp. black pepper
- 1 yellow squash, diced
- 1 onion, chopped

Directions:
Place a pan on medium heat and add olive oil to it. Put tomatoes, onion, garlic, oregano, black pepper, sugar, and basil. Cover it with the lid. Simmer for half an hour on low heat. Heat the broiler and put the grill away from the heat source. Grease the baking pan with cooking spray. Brush some olive oil over zucchini, peppers, and squash. Place them on the broiler and cook for eight minutes. Then keep it aside. Boil some water in a pot and cook the pasta in it. Once done, drain out the excess water. Mix the pasta with the sauce, top it up with vegetables, and then serve.
Nutrition: Calories 363; Fat 10g; Carbohydrates 65g; Proteins 12g; Cholesterol 0mg; Sodium 23mg

Pumpkin Pasta Sauce

Preparation time: 10 minutes **Cooking time:** 20 minutes **Servings:** 2
Ingredients:
- 2 c. pasta
- 2 tsp. olive oil
- 10 oz. pumpkin, pureed
- 8 oz. mushrooms
- 1 onion, chopped
- 2 garlic cloves, crushed
- 1 c. vegetable broth
- ½ tsp. sage
- 1/8 tsp. salt
- ¼ tsp. black pepper
- 1 Tbsp. parsley
- 1/4 c. Parmesan cheese

Directions:
Boil water in a pan and cook the pasta in it. Put another pan on medium flame. Add mushrooms, onion, and olive oil with garlic and sauté them for ten minutes. Pour the broth into the pan with sage, pumpkin puree, salt, and pepper. Simmer for eight minutes on low heat. Once the pasta is done, drain the excess water and put it in the pumpkin sauce. Stir it well. Garnish with Parmesan cheese and serve.
Nutrition: Calories 197; Fat 5g; Carbohydrates 29g; Proteins 9g; Cholesterol 4mg; Sodium 176mg

Vegan Bowl

Preparation time: 5 minutes **Cooking time:** 60 minutes **Servings:** 4
Ingredients:
- 1 c. brown Rice
- 2 tsp. canola oil
- 4 lime wedges
- 1 c. red onion
- 1 c. diced sweet potato
- Avocado halved
- 2 c. green bell pepper
- 1 chili pepper
- 2 garlic cloves, crushed
- 1 c. tomato, diced
- 1/2 c. green lentils
- 1/2 c. red lentils
- 1 Tbsp. cumin
- 1 Tbsp. pepper
- 1 Tbsp. red wine vinegar
- 2 c. vegetable stock
- 2 c. water
- 4 c. kale
- 1 c. black beans
- 2 Tbsp. fresh cilantro

Directions:
Take a large sauté pan and heat oil on medium to high heat. Add tomato, onion, sweet potato, garlic, and peppers. Cook the ingredients for 10 to 15 minutes or until the onions look translucent. After that, add vinegar, Rice, stock, spices, and water. Bring the ingredients to a boil and reduce to a simmer. Cover the sauté pan and cook for 40 to 45 minutes. For serving, toss the vegetables with black beans, cilantro, and avocado, and garnish with lime wedges. Serve immediately.
Nutrition: Calories 376; Fat 4g; Carbohydrates 68g; Proteins 18g; Cholesterol 0mg; Sodium 67mg

Halibut with Tomato Salsa

Preparation time: 10 mins **Cooking time:** 10-15 mins **Servings:** 2
Ingredients:
- 2 halibut Fillets
- 1 tomato
- 2 Tbsp. basil
- 1 tsp. oregano
- 1 Tbsp. garlic, crushed
- 2 tsp. olive oil

Directions:
Preheat the oven to 350 F. Take a 9x13-inch baking tray and coat it with cooking spray. Then take a small bowl and combine basil, garlic, tomato, and oregano. Mix the ingredients well by adding olive oil. Now, arrange the halibut Fillets in the baking tray and spoon the tomato mixture over them. Then bake the fish fillets for about 10-15 minutes. Immediately dish out your prepared delicious halibut fillets.
Nutrition: Calories 140; Fat 4g; Carbohydrates 4g; Proteins 22g; Cholesterol 55mg; Sodium 84mg.

Herb-Crust Cod

Preparation time: 15 minutes **Cooking time:** 10-15 minutes **Servings:** 2
Ingredients:
- 2 cod fillets
- 3/4 c. herb-flavored stuffing
- 2 Tbsp. honey

Directions:
For preparing the herb-crust cod, preheat the oven to 375°F and take a 9x13-inch baking tray and coat it with cooking spray. Take a bag, place stuffing in and seal it. Now crush the filling well until a crumbly texture is achieved. After that, brush the Fillets with honey and place them into the bag of stuffing. Gently shake the bag of Fillets so that the crumbs evenly coat the Fillets. Repeat the process with the remaining Fillets and place the cod Fillets over the baking tray. Bake the fish Fillets for about 10-15 minutes. Immediately dish out your prepared delicious cod Fillets.
Nutrition: Calories 150; Fat 1g; Carbohydrates 14g; Proteins 21g; Cholesterol 49mg; Sodium 158mg

Honey Crusted Chicken

Preparation time: 15 minutes **Cooking time:** 25 minutes **Servings:** 2
Ingredients:
- 2 chicken breasts
- 4 saltine crackers
- 4 tsp. honey
- 1 tsp. paprika

Directions:
Preheat the oven to 380° F and coat the baking tray with cooking spray. Then crush the crackers and place them in a small mixing bowl. Add paprika to crushed crackers and stir both ingredients to mix well. Add honey and chicken to another mixing bowl and toss them to coat evenly. Add in the cracker mixture and press the chicken in the mix until the chicken is evenly coated on both sides. Place the chicken breast pieces on the prepared baking tray and bake until it is lightly browned for about 20-25 minutes. Serve your honey-crusted chicken immediately.
Nutrition: Calories 224; Fat 4g; Carbohydrates 20g; Proteins 27g; Cholesterol 83mg; Sodium 204mg

Zucchini-Chickpea Burgers

Preparation time: 10 minutes **Cooking time:** 15 minutes **Servings:** 2
Ingredients:
- 3 tsp. miso
- 10 oz. chickpeas
- 4 whole grain buns
- 4 Tbsp. tahini
- ½ c. zucchini
- 1 Tbsp. lemon juice
- 2 tomatoes
- ¼ tsp. onion powder
- 1 c. arugula
- ¼ tsp. garlic
- ¼ tsp. pepper
- 2 Tbsp. water
- 1 tsp. chives
- 1 tsp. cumin
- ¼ tsp. salt
- ¼ c. parsley
- ⅓ c. oats
- 1 Tbsp. olive oil

Directions:
Take a bowl and mix all the spices with the tahini. Then add in the chives and keep them aside. Take a blender and blend the chickpeas with all the spices, including the tahini sauce. Make a smooth thick paste, toss chives with parsley, and blend again. Add the oats with the zucchini to the chickpea mix and combine them with your hands. Make patties of medium size. Heat oil in a pan and put the cakes in it.

Stir fry the patties for four minutes from both sides. Once done, put them on the buns with tomato slices, arugula, and ranch sauce. Cover the bun with another piece and serve.
Nutrition: Calories 373; Fat 15g; Carbohydrates 49g; Proteins 13g; Sodium 531mg; Potassium 522mg

Chicken Tenders with Bagel Seasoning

Preparation time: 10 minutes **Cooking time:** 15 minutes **Servings:** 2
Ingredients:
- 1 lb. chicken
- 1 egg
- 5 oz. greens
- ½ c. breadcrumbs
- 1 Tbsp. bagel seasoning
- 2 Tbsp. olive oil
- 1 Tbsp. vinegar
- 1 tsp. mustard
- 1 tsp. Honey
- ⅛ tsp. pepper

Directions:
Whisk the eggs in a bowl with bagel seasoning. Take the chicken, place it in the egg mix, and coat it with the breadcrumbs. In a pan, heat the olive oil. Cook the chicken in the oil for five minutes till it becomes golden. Now add in all the other ingredients and cook for another minute. Serve with the greens.
Nutrition: Calories 394; Fat 26g; Carbohydrates 14g; Proteins 27g; Cholesterol 110mg; Sodium 402mg; Potassium 338mg

Honey-Garlic Chicken Thighs

Preparation time: 5 minutes **Cooking time:** 20 minutes **Servings:** 2
Ingredients:
- 4 oz. chicken thighs
- ¼ c. honey
- 3 cloves garlic
- ½ tsp. pepper
- 1 Tbsp. canola oil
- ¾ c. water
- 1 Tbsp. Soy sauce
- ¼ tsp. salt
- 2 Tbsp. vinegar
- 2 Tbsp. butter
- 2 Tbsp. chives

Directions:
Set the oven to 425° Fahrenheit. Using paper towels, press the chicken dry and sprinkle thoroughly with spice. In a wide oven-safe pan, heat the oil on medium flame. Cook the chicken for ten minutes, until the skin is golden brown and crispy Transfer the chicken to the oven after flipping it and bake for fifteen minutes. Remove the pan from the oven, place it on a plate, and cover it with aluminum foil. Put a pan over medium flame. Heat a little oil and add chopped garlic and chives. Pour a little water while scrubbing the bottom of the pan to release bits of food. Simmer and stir constantly for four minutes until the liquid has decreased, and the garlic has softened. Then, add hot honey, soy sauce, salt, and water and cook until the sauce is thick enough to coat the back of a spoon for five minutes. Take it off the heat and whisk in vinegar and butter till melted. Put the chicken into the gravy and toss it over to cover it evenly. Serve and top with chives.
Nutrition: Calories 282; Fat 14g; Carbohydrates 20g; Proteins 22g; Cholesterol 111mg; Sodium 391mg; Potassium 301mg

Chapter 8: MEAT RECIPES

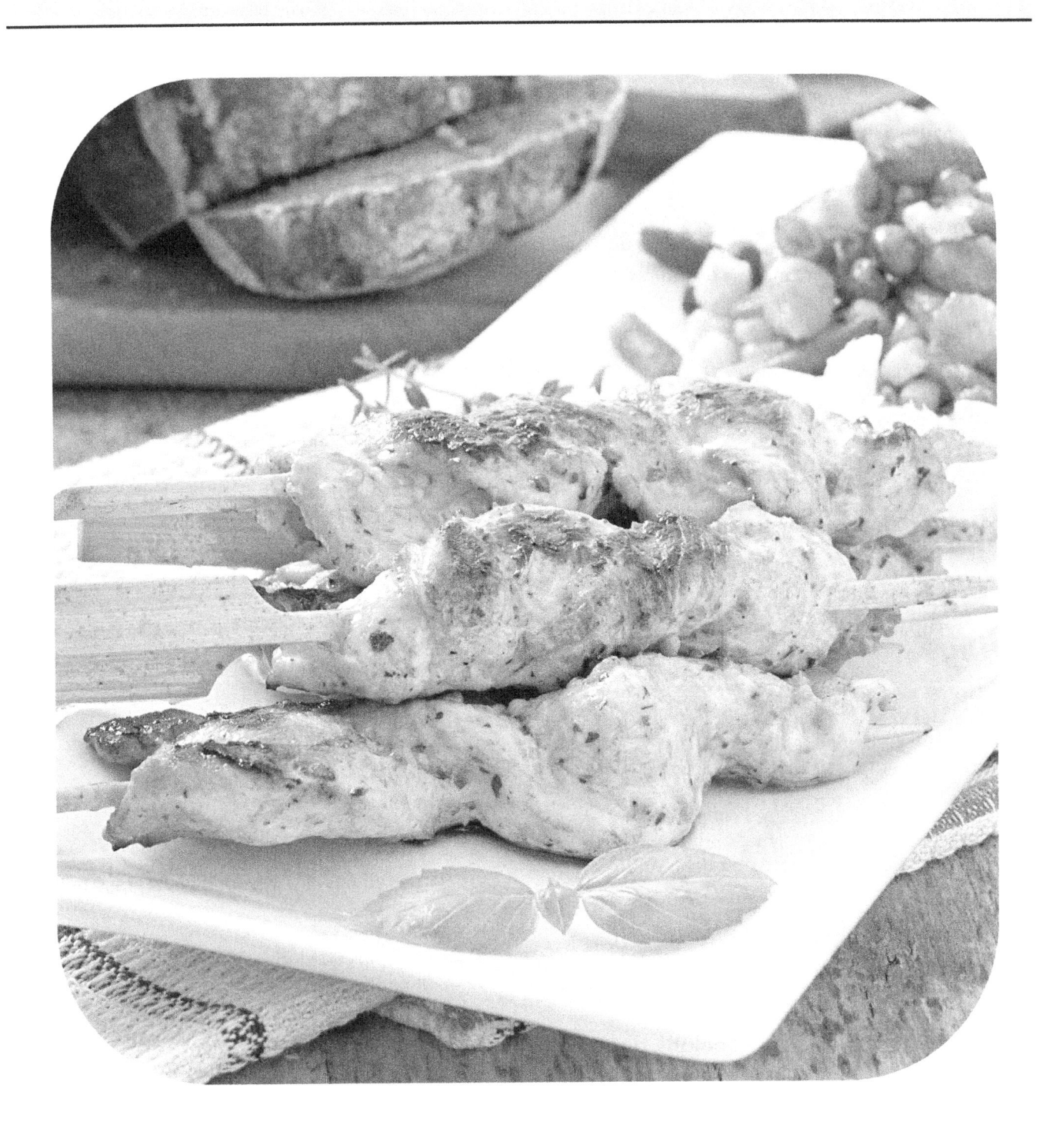

Spiced Beef

Preparation time: 10 minutes **Cooking time:** 80 minutes **Servings:** 2
Ingredients:
- 1-pound beef sirloin
- 1 tablespoon five-spice seasoning
- 1 bay leaf
- 2 cups of water
- 1 teaspoon peppercorn

Directions:
Place the meat in the pan after seasoning it with five spice. Peppercorns, water, and any leaf may be added. On medium heat, simmer it for 80 minutes with the lid on. Slice the cooked meat, then pour hot spiced water over it from the pan.
Nutrition: 213 Calories, 34.5g Protein, 0.5g Carbohydrates, 7.1g Fat, 0.2g Fiber, 101mg Cholesterol, 116mg Sodium, 466mg Potassium.

Tomato Beef

Preparation time: 10 minutes **Cooking time:** 17 minutes **Servings:** 2
Ingredients:
- 2 chuck shoulder steaks
- ¼ cup tomato sauce
- 1 tablespoon olive oil

Directions:
Brush the steaks with tomato sauce and olive oil and transfer to the preheated 390F grill. Grill the meat for 9 minutes. Then flip it to another side and cook for 8 minutes more.
Nutrition: 247 Calories, 21.4g Protein, 1.7g Carbohydrates, 17.1g Fat, 0.5g Fiber, 70mg Cholesterol, 231mg Sodium, 101mg Potassium.

Beef Tenderloin Medallions With Yogurt Sauce

Preparation time: 10 minutes **Cooking time:** 5 minutes **Serves** 4
Ingredients:
For the horseradish sauce
- ¾ cup whole-milk Greek yogurt
- 2 tablespoons prepared horseradish
- 1 garlic clove, minced
- ¼ teaspoon freshly ground black pepper
- 2 teaspoons 1% milk

For the medallions
- 12 ounces beef tenderloin, flattened and cut into 4 pieces
- ½ teaspoon freshly ground black pepper
- ½ teaspoon garlic powder
- 1 tablespoon unsalted butter

Direction:
To make the horseradish sauce
Whisk together the yogurt, horseradish, garlic, pepper, and milk in a small bowl until well-mixed. Divide the sauce among 4 condiment cups.
To make the medallions.
Season the tenderloin with pepper and garlic powder. In a large skillet, melt the butter over medium-high heat. Add the beef and sauté for about 2 minutes on each side, until the outside is browned and the inside is very pink, medium-rare. Remove from the heat. When cool, portion the beef into 4 storage containers. To serve, reheat the meat and top with horseradish sauce.
Nutrition: Calories: 185; Total fat: 9g; Carbohydrates: 3g; Fiber: 0.5g; Protein: 23g; Calcium: 72mg; Vitamin D: 3 IU; Potassium: 332mg; Magnesium: 18mg; Sodium: 87m

Mustardy Zucchini Beef Burger

Preparation time: 15 minutes **Cooking time:** 10 minutes **Serves** 4
Ingredients:
- ½ cup cooked pinto beans
- ½ cup minced onion
- ½ cup minced mushrooms
- ½ cup finely chopped red bell pepper
- 1 medium carrot, grated
- 1 medium zucchini, grated
- 2 cloves garlic, minced
- ¾ pound 94% lean ground beef (grass-fed if possible)
- 1 tablespoon ground mustard
- ½ cup shredded low-fat cheddar cheese
- Salt and freshly ground black pepper
- 1 tablespoon extra-virgin olive oil
- Lettuce leaves or whole-wheat buns
- Optional toppings: avocado slices, tomato slices, fresh parsley

Direction:
In a large bowl, gently mash the beans with the back of a large spoon. Add the onion, mushrooms, bell pepper, carrot, zucchini, garlic, beef, mustard, cheddar, and a dash each of salt and pepper and combine well. Form into 4 patties. In a large skillet, heat the olive oil over medium-high heat. Add the patties and sear them until dark brown on one side,

about 5 minutes. Flip and cook for another 5 minutes or until your desired doneness. Serve the burgers on lettuce leaves or toasted buns. Garnish with optional toppings, if desired.
Nutrition: Calories: 226 | Fat: 9g | Protein: 24g | Carbohydrates: 12g| Fiber: 4g | Sugar: 3g| Sodium: 140mg

Garlicky Beef Tenderloin with Artichoke

Preparation time: 10 minutes **Cooking time:** 15 minutes **Serves** 4
Ingredients:
- 1 tablespoon extra-virgin olive oil
- 4 beef tenderloin filets (4 ounces each), trimmed of fat
- 4 cloves garlic, chopped
- Pinch of red pepper flakes
- 4 cups of baby spinach
- 1 (15-ounce) can of chickpeas, rinsed and drained
- 1 (14-ounce) can of water-packed artichoke hearts, drained and rinsed
- 1 cup chopped fresh tomatoes, with their juices
- 2 teaspoons dried marjoram
- ½ cup chopped fresh basil leaves
- Salt and freshly ground black pepper (optional)

Direction:
In a large sauté pan, heat the olive oil over medium-high heat until shimmering. Add the beef and cook until the filets are well browned on the bottom, about 2 minutes. Flip and cook until well browned on the second side, another 2 minutes. Transfer to a plate and cover to keep warm. Reduce the heat under the skillet to medium. Add the garlic and sauté until golden brown, about 1 minute. Add the pepper flakes and spinach. Cook and stir for 1 minute to wilt the spinach. Add ½ cup water, cover the pan and bring to a simmer. Uncover and cook until almost all the water is evaporated, 3 to 4 minutes. Add chickpeas, artichoke hearts, tomatoes with their juices, and marjoram. Cook for 2 minutes and stir until the sauce coats the vegetables. Return the beef to the pan and any collected juices on the plate and toss the fresh basil. Cover and cook until the meat is cooked to your desired doneness, 2 to 3 minutes. Place a beef filet on each of 4 serving plates. Season the vegetables with salt and pepper, if desired, and portion onto the plates with the beef.
Nutrition: Calories: 348| Fat: 11g | Protein: 34g | Carbohydrates: 29g| Fiber: 12g | Sugar: 4g| Sodium: 129mg

Beef with Spicy Vegetable Stir-Fry

Preparation time: 15 minutes **Cooking time:** 12 minutes **Serves** 2
Ingredients:
- ¾ cup orange juice
- 1 tablespoon reduced-sodium soy sauce
- 1 tablespoon unseasoned rice vinegar or dry sherry
- 1 teaspoon sesame oil
- 2 teaspoons corn starch
- ¼ teaspoon Chinese five-spice powder
- 1 teaspoon red pepper flakes
- 2 teaspoons extra-virgin olive oil
- 8 ounces boneless beef sirloin steak, cut into thin strips
- 3 cloves garlic, minced
- 2 teaspoons grated fresh ginger
- 3 cups frozen stir-fry vegetable blend

Direction:
In a small bowl, combine the orange juice, soy sauce, rice vinegar, sesame oil, cornstarch, five-spice, and pepper flakes until smooth. Set aside. In a large skillet or wok, heat 1 teaspoon of the olive oil over high heat. Add the beef and stir-fry until no longer pink, 3 to 4 minutes. Remove with a slotted spoon to a plate; cover to keep warm. Add the remaining 1 teaspoon of olive oil to the pan. Add the garlic and ginger and stir-fry for 1 minute. Add the vegetables and continue cooking for 2 to 3 minutes until thawed. Stir the sauce and pour into the pan, bring to a boil, and cook for 2 to 3 minutes to thicken. Return the beef to the pan, stir to combine, and cook for 1 to 2 minutes to heat through.
Nutrition: Calories: 321 | Fat: 12g | Protein: 28g | Carbohydrates: 22g| Fiber: 4g | Sugar: 13g| Sodium: 376mg

Beef Tenderloin with Balsamic Tomatoes

Preparation Time: 5 Minutes **Cooking Time:** 20 Minutes **Serves** 2
Ingredients:
- ½ cup balsamic vinegar
- ¾ cup coarsely chopped, seeded tomato
- 2 teaspoons olive oil
- 2 (3- to 4-ounce, ¾-inch-thick) beef tenderloin steaks, trimmed of visible fat

- 1 teaspoon fresh thyme (or ½ teaspoon dried)

Direction:
Bring the balsamic vinegar to a boil in a small saucepan. The liquid should be reduced to 1/4 cup after 5 minutes of simmering, uncovered. Add the tomatoes and simmer for a further one to two minutes. Turn off the heat and remove the pot. Olive oil should be heated to a medium-high temperature in a big skillet. Turn down the heat to medium, then add the steaks. Turn the steaks once when cooking it to the desired doneness. Allow 7 to 9 minutes for medium (160°F) on each side. Add the thyme after spooning the balsamic tomatoes over the steaks. Serve right away.
Nutrition: Calories: 298; Total Fat: 20g; Saturated Fat: 7g; Cholesterol: 58mg; Sodium: 69mg; Potassium: 407mg; Magnesium: 24mg; Total Carbohydrates: 11g; Fiber: 1g; Sugars: 0g; Protein: 17g

Fajita-Style Beef Tacos

Preparation Time: 5 Minutes **Cooking Time:** 15 Minutes **Serves** 4
Ingredients:
- 1 tablespoon olive oil
- 1 red bell pepper, sliced and deseeded
- 1 medium red onion, sliced
- 12 ounces flank steak, trimmed of fat, cut into thin strips
- ½ teaspoon chili powder
- 1 teaspoon cumin
- 8 (6-inch) whole-wheat flour tortillas, warmed
- 1 avocado, peeled, seeded, and cubed
- ¼ cup fresh cilantro
- ¼ cup feta cheese
- 4 lime wedges (optional)

Direction:
Heat the olive oil in a large skillet over medium-high heat for about 2 minutes. Add the bell peppers and onion and cook, often stirring, until just tender, about 5 minutes. Remove the vegetables from the skillet. Add the steak slices to the same skillet. Stir-fry for 2 to 3 minutes, or until no longer raw. Return the vegetables to the skillet, add the chili powder and cumin, and stir-fry for 2 to 3 minutes or until heated. Spoon the fajita filling into warm tortillas, and top with equal portions of avocado, cilantro, and a sprinkle of feta. Serve immediately with fresh limes (if using).
Nutrition: Calories: 456; Total Fat: 23g; Saturated Fat: 6g; Cholesterol: 35mg; Sodium: 745mg; Potassium: 560mg; Total Carbohydrates: 37g; Fiber: 21g; Sugars: 3g; Protein: 36g

One-Pot Spinach Beef Soup

Preparation Time: 15 minutes **Cooking Time:** 20 minutes **Servings:** 1
Ingredients:
- 1 pound of ground beef
- 3 garlic cloves, minced
- 2 cartons (32 ounces each) of reduced-sodium beef broth
- 2 cans (14-1/2 ounces each) diced tomatoes with green pepper, celery, and onion, undrained
- 1 teaspoon dried basil
- 1/2 teaspoon pepper
- 4 cups fresh spinach, coarsely chopped
- Grated Parmesan cheese
- 1/2 teaspoon dried oregano
- 1/4 teaspoon salt
- 3 cups uncooked bow tie pasta

Directions:
Cook beef and garlic in a 6-quart stockpot over medium heat until meat is no longer pink, 6-8 minutes; crumble beef; drain. Bring broth, tomatoes, and spices to a boil. Return to a spot after adding the pasta. Cook uncovered, for 7-9 minutes, or until pasta is cooked. Stir in the spinach until it is wilted. Serve with cheese on top.
Nutrition: Calories: 321| Fat: 10g | Protein: 37g | Carbohydrates: 26g| Fiber: 12g | Sugar: 4g| Sodium: 129mg

Sesame Beef Skewers

Preparation Time: 15 minutes **Cooking Time:** 20 minutes **Servings:** 1
Ingredients:
- 1 pound beef top sirloin steak
- 6 tablespoons sesame ginger salad dressing, divided
- 1 tablespoon reduced-sodium soy sauce
- 1/4 teaspoon pepper
- 1 tablespoon sesame seed, toasted
- 2 cups chopped fresh pineapple
- 2 medium apples, chopped
- 1 tablespoon sweet chili sauce
- 1 tablespoon lime juice

Directions:
Toss beef with three tablespoons of dressing and soy sauce in a mixing basin; set aside for 10 minutes. Meanwhile, stir pineapple, apples, chili sauce, lime juice, and pepper in a large mixing bowl. Thread

steak onto four moistened wooden or metal skewers; remove leftover marinade. Grill kabobs, covered, over medium heat for 7-9 minutes, rotating periodically; brush generously with remaining dressing during the last 3 minutes. Sesame seeds are optional. With the pineapple combination, serve.
Nutrition: Calories: 311| Fat: 10g | Protein: 34g | Carbohydrates: 27g| Fiber: 12g | Sugar: 4g| Sodium: 122mg

Best Lasagna Soup

Preparation Time: 15 minutes **Cooking Time:** 20 minutes **Servings:** 1
Ingredients:
- 1-pound lean ground beef (90% lean)
- 1 large green pepper, chopped
- 1 medium onion, chopped
- 2 garlic cloves, minced
- 2 cans (14-1/2 ounces each) diced tomatoes, undrained
- 1/4 teaspoon pepper
- 2-1/2 cups uncooked spiral pasta
- 1/2 cup shredded Parmesan cheese
- 2 cans (14-1/2 ounces each) of reduced-sodium beef broth
- 1 can (8 ounces) tomato sauce
- 1 cup frozen corn
- 1/4 cup tomato paste
- 2 teaspoons Italian seasoning

Directions:
Cook beef, green pepper, and onion in a large saucepan over medium heat for 6-8 minutes, or until the meat are no longer pink, breaking up the steak into crumbles. Cook for 1 minute more after adding the garlic. Drain. Combine the tomatoes, broth, tomato sauce, corn, tomato paste, Italian seasoning, and pepper in a mixing bowl. Bring the water to a boil. Mix in the pasta. Bring back to a spot. Reduce heat to low and cover for 10-12 minutes, or until tender pasta. Garnish with cheese.
Nutrition: Calories: 322| Fat: 11g | Protein: 33g | Carbohydrates: 29g| Fiber: 10g | Sugar: 4g| Sodium: 115 mg

Chapter 9: fish and seafood recipes

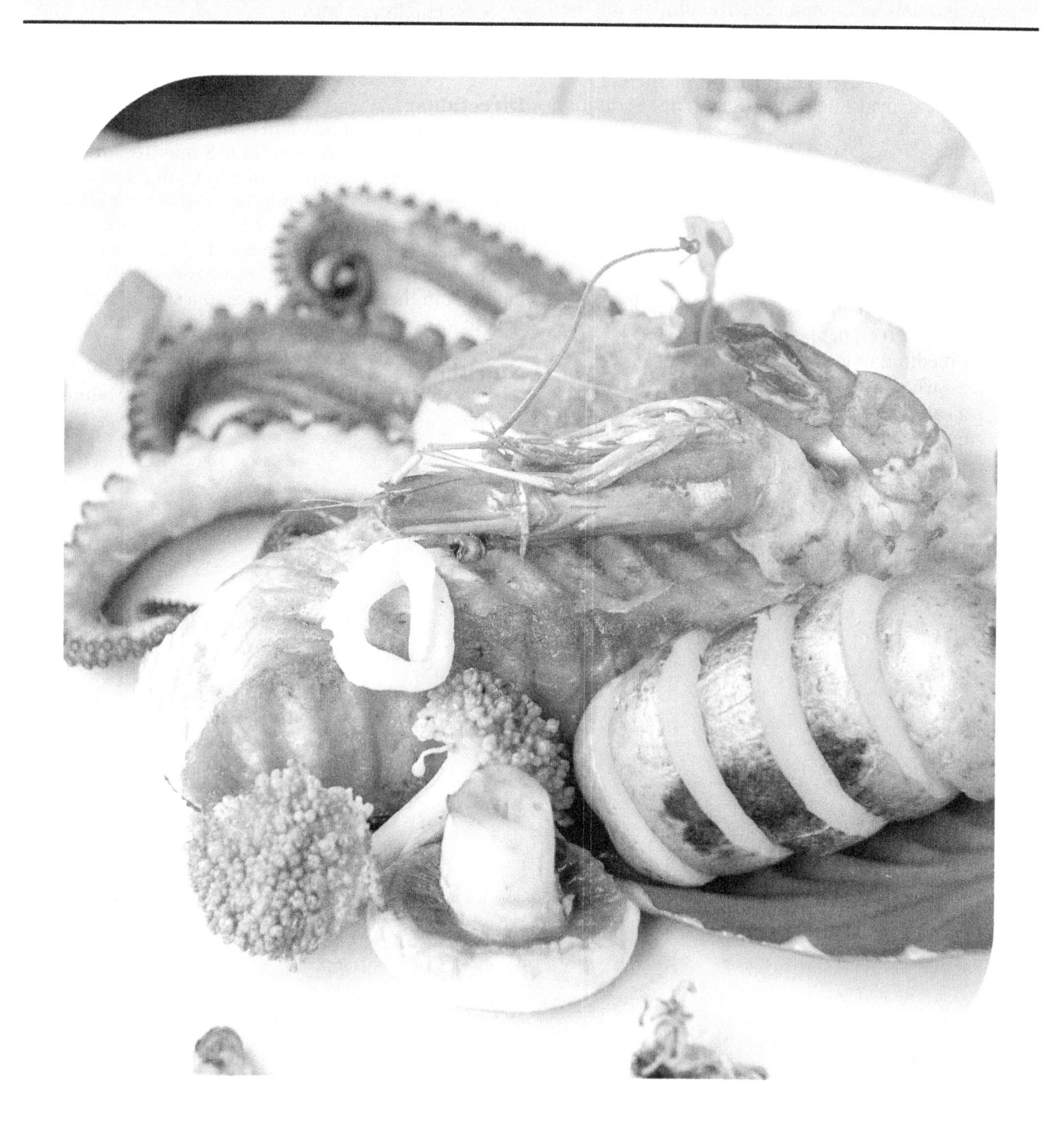

Catfish with Egg Pecans

Preparation time: 10 minutes **Cooking time:** 20 minutes **Serves** 4
Ingredients:
- 4 catfish fillets (approximately 1 pound)
- ½ teaspoon freshly ground black pepper
- ½ teaspoon garlic powder
- 2 teaspoons dried rosemary
- 2 egg whites, beaten
- ¾ cup pecans, chopped
- Lemon wedges for serving

Direction:
Preheat the oven to 400°F. Line a baking sheet with foil and coat the foil with nonstick cooking spray. Sprinkle the catfish fillets with the black pepper, garlic, and rosemary, then dip each fillet into the egg whites to coat. Place the chopped pecans on a plate and press the egg-coated fillets firmly into the pecans, turning to coat both sides. Place the fillets on the baking sheet. Bake for 20 minutes or until the fish flakes easily with a fork. Serve with lemon wedges and enjoy.
Nutrition: Calories: 263 | Fat: 2g | Protein: 18g | Carbohydrates: 4g| Fiber: 3g | Sugar: 1g| Sodium: 228mg

Roast Salmon with Tarragon

Preparation time: 10 minutes **Cooking time:** 15 minutes **Serves** 2
Ingredients:
- 2 (5-ounce) salmon fillets with skin
- 2 teaspoons olive oil, plus extra for drizzling
- Salt
- Freshly ground black pepper
- 1 bunch asparagus, trimmed
- 1 teaspoon dried chives
- 1 teaspoon dried tarragon
- Fresh lemon wedges for serving

Direction:
Preheat the oven to 425°F. Rub salmon all over with 1 teaspoon of olive oil per fillet. Season with salt and pepper. Place asparagus spears on a foil-lined baking sheet and lay the salmon fillets skin-side down on top. Place the pan in the upper third of the oven and roast for 12 minutes, or until the fish is just cooked. Roasting time will vary depending on the thickness of your salmon. Salmon should flake easily with a fork when ready, and an instant-read thermometer should register 145°F. When cooked, remove from the oven, cut fillets in half crosswise, then lift flesh from skin with a spatula and transfer to a plate. Discard the skin, drizzle salmon with oil, sprinkle with herbs, and serve with lemon wedges and roasted asparagus spears.
Nutrition: Calories: 353 | Fat: 22g | Protein: 34g | Carbohydrates: 5g| Fiber: 2g | Sugar: 0g| Sodium: 90mg

Pasta with Lemon Spiced Shrimp and Cheese

Preparation time: 10 minutes **Cooking time:** 15 minutes **Serves** 2
Ingredients:
- 2 tablespoons olive oil
- 1 tablespoon garlic, minced
- 2 cups assorted fresh vegetables
- 4 ounces frozen shrimp, cooked, peeled, and deveined
- Salt Freshly ground black pepper
- Juice of ½ lemon
- 4 ounces whole-wheat angel-hair pasta,
- 2 tablespoons grated Parmesan cheese

Direction:
Heat the oil in a large nonstick skillet over medium heat. Add the garlic and sauté for 1 minute. Add vegetables and sauté until crisp-tender, 3 to 4 minutes. Add the shrimp and sauté until just heated through. Season lightly with salt and pepper, and squeeze lemon juice over the shrimp and vegetables. Continue to cook for about 2 minutes until the fluids have been reduced by almost half. Remove from heat. Toss shrimp and vegetables with pasta. Serve topped with Parmesan cheese.
Nutrition: Calories: 439 | Fat: 17g | Protein: 23g | Carbohydrates: 50g| Fiber: 8g | Sugar: 5g| Sodium: 286mg

Tomatoes with Tilapia Tacos

Preparation time: 10 minutes **Cooking time:** 10 minutes **Serves** 4
Ingredients:
- 1 teaspoon olive oil
- 1 pound tilapia fillets
- 3 cups diced tomatoes
- ½ cup fresh cilantro, chopped
- 3 tablespoons lime juice
- Salt
- Freshly ground black pepper
- 8 (5-inch) white-corn tortillas
- 1 avocado sliced into 8 wedges
- Optional: lime wedges and fat-free sour cream for serving

Direction:
Heat the oil in a large skillet, add the tilapia and cook until the flesh starts to flake, about 5 minutes per side. Add the tomatoes, cilantro, and lime juice. Sauté over medium-high heat for about 5 minutes, breaking up the fish to get everything mixed well. Season to taste with salt and pepper. Meanwhile, heat tortillas on a skillet for a few minutes on each side to warm. Serve ¼ cup of fish mixture on each warmed tortilla with two slices of avocado. Serve immediately with optional toppings if using.
Nutrition: Calories: 286 | Fat: 12g | Protein: 28g | Carbohydrates: 22g| Fiber: 4g | Sugar: 0g| Sodium: 117mg

Garlic-Baked Flounder

Preparation time: 10 minutes **Cooking time:** 15 minutes **Serves** 2
Ingredients:
- 14 Brussels sprouts
- 2 tablespoons olive oil
- 3 tablespoons lemon juice
- 1 tablespoon minced fresh garlic
- ¼ teaspoon dried dill
- 2 (6-ounce) flounder fillets
- Salt
- Freshly ground black pepper

Direction:
Preheat the oven to 400°F. Rinse the Brussels sprouts and pat them dry. Cut their stem ends, cut shoots in half, and place them on a foil-lined baking pan. Drizzle with 1 tablespoon olive oil and toss to coat. Meanwhile, stir together 1 tablespoon of olive oil, lemon juice, garlic, and dill in a small bowl. Rinse flounder fillets and pat dry. Season lightly with salt and pepper. Place the baking dish evenly and drizzle the oil-and-herb mixture over flounder fillets. Bake for 10 to 11 minutes, or until the fish flakes easily when tested with a fork. The Brussels sprouts should be lightly browned and pierce easily with a fork. Divide the flounder and Brussels sprouts between serving plates.
Nutrition: Calories: 319 | Fat: 17g | Protein: 33g | Carbohydrates: 13g| Fiber: 5g | Sugar: 3g| Sodium: 529mg

Seafood Dip

Preparation Time: 10 minutes **Cooking Time:** 30 minutes **Servings:** 16
Ingredients:
- 1/2 lb. shrimp, cooked
- 4 oz can green chilies
- 2 cups pepper jack cheddar
- 4 oz cream cheddar
- 1/2 tsp old straight flavoring
- 2 garlic cloves, minced
- 1/2 cup spinach, minced
- 1/2 cup onion, minced
- 2 tbsp margarine
- 4 oz crab meat

Directions:
Preheat the broiler to 425° F. Melt margarine in a skillet over medium intensity. Add garlic, old narrows preparing, spinach, crab meat, chilies, and shrimp, and cook for 4-5 minutes. Add 1 cup pepper jack cheddar and cream cheddar. Top with residual cheddar and prepare for 20 minutes. Servings and appreciation.
Nutrition: Calories 63 •Fat 4 g •Carbs 1 g •Sugar 0.2 g •Protein 5 g •Cholesterol 45 mg

Spinach Shrimp Alfredo

Preparation Time: 10 minutes **Cooking Time:** 15 minutes **Servings:** 2
Ingredients:
- 1/2 lb. shrimp, deveined
- 2 garlic cloves, minced
- 2 tbsp onion, cleaved
- 1 cup new spinach, cleaved
- 1/2 cup weighty cream
- 1 tbsp spread
- Pepper
- Salt

Directions:
Melt spread in a skillet over medium intensity. Add onion, garlic, and shrimp to the container and sauté for 3 minutes. Add leftover ingredients and stew for 7 minutes or until cooked. Servings and appreciation.
Nutrition: Calories 300 •Fat 19 g •Starches 5 g • Sugar 0.5 g •Protein 27 g •Cholesterol 295 mg

Shrimp Scampi

Preparation Time: 10 minutes **Cooking Time:** 10 minutes **Servings:** 4
Ingredients:
- 1 lb. shrimp
- 1/4 tsp red pepper pieces
- 1 tbsp new lemon juice
- 1/4 cup margarine
- 1/2 cup chicken stock
- 2 garlic cloves, minced

- 1 shallot, cut
- 3 tbsp olive oil
- 3 tbsp parsley, cleaved
- Pepper
- Salt

Directions:
Heat oil in a container over medium intensity. Add garlic and shallots and cook for 3 minutes. Add stock, lemon squeeze, and margarine, and cook for 5 minutes. Add red pepper chips, parsley, pepper, and salt. Mix. Add shrimp and cook for 3 minutes. Servings and appreciation.
Nutrition: Calories 336 •Fat 24 g •Carbs 3 g •Sugar 0.2 g •Protein 26 g •Cholesterol 269 mg

Fish Salad

Preparation Time: 5 minutes **Cooking Time:** 5 minutes **Servings:** 2
Ingredients:
- 5 oz can fish, depleted
- 1 tsp Dijon mustard
- 2 tbsp dill pickles, cleaved
- 1 tbsp new chives, cleaved
- 2 tbsp mayonnaise
- Pepper
- Salt

Directions:
Add all ingredients into the giant bowl and blend well. 2.Servings and appreciation.
Nutrition: Calories 143 •Fat 5.6 g •Carbs 4 g •Sugar 1 g •Protein 18 g •Cholesterol 25 mg

Flavors Shrimp Scampi

Preparation Time: 10 minutes **Cooking Time:** 25 minutes **Servings:** 4
Ingredients:
- 1 lb. shrimp, stripped and deveined
- 4 tbsp parmesan cheddar, ground
- 1 cup chicken stock
- 1 tbsp garlic, minced
- 1/2 cup spread

Directions:
Preheat the stove to 350° F. Melt spread in a pot over medium intensity. Add garlic and sauté for a minute. Add stock and mix well. Add shrimp to the glass dish and pour spread blend over the shrimp. Top with ground cheddar and prepare for 10-12 minutes. Servings and appreciation.
Nutrition: Calories 388 •Fat 27 g •Carbs 2.7 g •Sugar 0.2 g •Protein 30.4 g •Cholesterol 307 mg

Creamy Tuna Salad

Preparation Time: 10 Minutes **Cooking Time:** 0 minutes **Serves:** 2
Ingredients:
- 1 (5 oz) can of water-packed tuna, drained
- 1 large, ripe avocado, pitted, peeled, and mashed
- 2 spring onions, finely chopped
- ½ lime, juiced
- 2 tbsp avocado oil
- ¼ tsp acceptable sea salt
- ¼ tsp ground black pepper
- 4 whole-wheat bread slices

Directions:
Add the drained tuna, mashed avocado, chopped spring onion, lime juice, avocado oil, acceptable sea salt, and ground black pepper in a small mixing bowl. Mix until well combined. Spoon the avocado mixture equally between 2 slices of bread, and top with the remaining two slices. Serve cold.
Nutrition: Calories: 518; Total Fat: 32g; Saturated Fat: 5g; Sodium: 567mg; Total Carbs: 41g; Fiber: 13g; Protein: 23g

Citrus Tilapia

Preparation time: 10 minutes **Cooking Time:** 25 Minutes **Serves:** 2
Ingredients:
- Aluminum foil
- 2 tbsp garlic, minced
- 2 rosemary sprigs, stems removed, chopped
- 1 oregano sprig, stem removed, chopped
- 2 tbsp olive oil
- 2 tilapia filets, cleaned and rinsed
- 2 lemons, sliced and divided
- 2 limes, sliced and divided
- ¼ tsp acceptable sea salt
- ¼ tsp ground black pepper

Directions:
Heat the oven to 450ºF, gas mark 8. Line a baking sheet with aluminum foil. Add the minced garlic, chopped rosemary, chopped oregano, and olive oil to a medium-sized mixing bowl. Mix to combine. Add the tilapia fillets to the bowl and coat generously with the olive oil mixture. Place the fillets on the prepared baking sheet. Place half the lemon and lime slices on the fillets and season with acceptable sea salt and ground black pepper. Place the baking sheet in the oven, and bake for 18 to 22 minutes or until the fillets are cooked. Remove from the oven. Garnish with the

remaining lemon and lime slices and serve with your choice of side.
Nutrition: Calories: 218; Total Fat: 3g; Saturated Fat: 1g; Sodium: 430mg; Total Carbs: 0g; Fiber: 0g; Protein: 45g

Lebanese-style cod fillets

Preparation time: 5 minutes **Cooking Time:** 15 Minutes **Serves:** 4
Ingredients:
- Aluminum foil
- 4 (4 oz) cod fillets
- 2 tbsp olive oil
- 1 tsp za'atar
- ½ tsp acceptable sea salt
- ¼ tsp ground black pepper
- 1 lime, cut into wedges
- 2 tbsp cilantro, finely chopped

Directions:
Heat the oven to 400°F, gas mark 6. Line a baking sheet with aluminum foil. Place the cod fillets on the baking sheet, and drizzle with olive oil. Season both sides of the fillets with za'atar, acceptable sea salt, and ground black pepper. Place the baking sheet in the oven, and bake for 6 to 8 minutes. Flip, and cook for 5 more minutes, or until the fillets flake easily with a fork. Remove from the oven. Serve the fillets topped with lime wedges and chopped cilantro.
Nutrition: Calories: 164; Total Fat: 8g; Saturated Fat: 1g; Sodium: 369mg; Total Carbs: 0g; Fiber: 0g; Protein: 21g

Salmon Sage Bake

Preparation time: 5 minutes **Cooking time:** 15 minutes **Serves:** 2
Ingredients:
- Aluminum foil
- 10 broccoli florets
- ¼ tsp ground black pepper
- 1 lime, divided
- 2 (4 oz) salmon fillets, skin removed
- 2 tbsp whole-grain mustard
- ¼ cup sage, finely chopped

Directions:
Heat the oven to 375°F, gas mark 5. Line a baking sheet with aluminum foil. Place broccoli florets on the baking sheet and season with ground black pepper. Divide the broccoli into two beds; five florets for each fish. Cut the lime in half, and cut one half into slices. Reserve the other half of the lime for after cooking. Place the lime slices on top of the broccoli florets, then place the salmon fillets on top of the limes. Add the whole-grain mustard and chopped sage to a small mixing bowl. Mix to combine. Evenly spread the mustard mixture on top of each salmon fillet. Cook for 15 minutes until the fish becomes opaque and flakes easily with a fork. Squeeze the lime juice from the reserved lime half onto both fillets, and serve warm.
Nutrition: Calories: 171, Total Fat: 5g, Saturated Fat: 2g, Cholesterol: 55mg, Sodium: 76mg, Total Carbs: 6g, Net Carbs: 4g, Fiber: 3g, Protein: 24g

Pine Nut Haddock

Preparation time: 5 minutes **Cooking time:** 15 minutes **Serves:** 2
Ingredients:
- Aluminum foil
- ½ cup cilantro, roughly chopped
- ¼ cup pine nuts
- ¼ tsp ground cumin
- ¼ tsp ground black pepper
- 2 tsp olive oil
- 1 large orange, zested and cut in half
- 2 (4 oz) haddock fillets, skin removed

Directions:
Heat the oven to 375°F, gas mark 5. Line a baking sheet with aluminum foil. In a food processor, combine the cilantro, pine nuts, ground cumin, ground black pepper, olive oil, and orange zest, and pulse until fine and incorporated. Cut one half of the orange into 4 slices. Place 2 orange slices on the baking sheet, overlapping each other, then place the haddock fillet on top. Repeat with the remaining orange slices and fish fillet. Spread 1½ tbsp of the pine nut mixture on each haddock fillet. Squeeze the juice from the other half of the orange on top. Bake for 10 to 12 minutes, until the haddock fillets flake easily with a fork. Serve warm.
Nutrition: Calories: 294, Total Fat: 21g, Saturated Fat: 3g, Cholesterol: 56mg, Sodium: 40mg, Total Carbs: 11g, Net Carbs: 7g, Fiber: 3g, Protein: 19g

Catalán Salmon Tacos

Preparation time: 10 minutes **Cooking time:** 20 minutes **Serves** 4
Ingredients:
- 1 teaspoon olive oil
- 1 (6-ounce) salmon fillet
- 1 teaspoon chili powder
- ½ teaspoon dried oregano leaves
- ⅛ teaspoon black pepper
- 1 small onion, diced

- 2 cloves peeled garlic, minced
- 1 (16-ounce) can of low-sodium white beans, rinsed and drained
- 1 tomato, chopped
- 1 cup torn fresh Swiss chard leaves
- 2 tablespoons pine nuts
- 4 corn tortillas, heated

Direction:
Add the olive oil to a large nonstick skillet and place over medium heat. Rub the salmon fillet with the chili powder, oregano, and pepper. Add the salmon to the pan, skin side down. Cook for 3 minutes, then turn and cook for 5 minutes longer, or until the fish flakes when tested with a fork. Remove the salmon from the pan, flake, and set aside. Add the onion and garlic to the pan and cook for 2 to 3 minutes, stirring, until softened. Add the beans and mash some of them into the onions. Cook for 1 minute, stirring occasionally. Add the tomato and Swiss chard and cook for another 1 to 2 minutes until the greens wilt. Add the pine nuts to the mixture. Make the tacos by adding the bean mixture and the salmon to the corn tortillas and folding them in half. Serve immediately.
Nutrition: Calories 296; Fat 8g (with 24% calories from fat); Saturated fat 1g; Monounsaturated fat 3g; Carbs 39g; Sodium 63mg; Protein 19g; Cholesterol 23mg; Sugar 2g

Salmon with Farro Pilaf

Preparation time: 5 minutes **Cooking time:** 25 minutes **Serves** 4
Ingredients:
- ½ cup farro
- 1¼ cups low-sodium vegetable broth
- 4 (4-ounce) salmon fillets
- Pinch salt
- ½ teaspoon dried marjoram leaves
- ⅛ teaspoon white pepper
- ¼ cup dried cherries
- ¼ cup dried currants
- 1 cup fresh baby spinach leaves
- 1 tablespoon orange juice

Direction:
Preheat the oven to 400°F. Line a baking sheet with parchment paper and set it aside. In a medium saucepan over medium heat, combine the farro and the vegetable broth and bring to a simmer. Reduce the heat to low and simmer, partially covered, for 25 minutes, or until the farro is tender. Meanwhile, sprinkle the salmon with the salt, marjoram, and white pepper and place it on the prepared baking sheet. When the farro has cooked for 10 minutes, bake the salmon in the oven for 12 to 15 minutes, or until the salmon flakes when tested with a fork. Remove and cover to keep warm. When the farro is tender, add the cherries, currants, spinach, and orange juice; stir and cover. Let stand off the heat for 2 to 3 minutes. Plate the salmon and serve with the farro pilaf.
Nutrition: Calories 304; Fat 8g ; Saturated fat 1g; Monounsaturated fat 2g; Carbs 32g; Sodium 139mg;; Protein 26g; Cholesterol 62mg; Sugar 17g

Salmon and Cauliflower Sheet Pan

Preparation time: 5 minutes, plus 30 minutes to marinate **Cooking time:** 20 minutes. **Serves** 4
Ingredients:
- 1 pound salmon fillet
- 3 tablespoons minced garlic, divided
- 2 tablespoons olive oil, divided
- 2 tablespoons low-sodium soy sauce
- Freshly ground black pepper
- 2½ cups bite-size cauliflower florets
- Pinch sea salt
- 1½ tablespoons maple syrup

Direction:
Place the salmon, 2 tablespoons garlic, 1 tablespoon oil, soy sauce, and pepper in a resealable plastic bag and place the bag in the refrigerator. Let the fish marinate for 30 minutes or overnight. Preheat the oven to 425°F. Line a baking sheet with parchment paper. In a medium bowl, toss the cauliflower with the remaining olive oil, garlic, more pepper, and a pinch of salt, and place it on half the prepared baking sheet. Place the marinated salmon on the other half of the sheet and bake for 20 minutes until the fish is slightly golden brown on the edges and just cooked through. Transfer the fish from the baking sheet to a plate and loosely cover it with foil to keep it warm. Flip the cauliflower and bake for 10 minutes more, until soft. Drizzle the maple syrup over the salmon and serve with the cauliflower.
Nutrition: Calories: 216; Total fat: 11g; Saturated fat: 2g; Trans fat: 0g; Protein: 20g; Total carbohydrate: 9g; Fiber: 1g; Sodium: 293mg; Potassium: 658mg

Spicy Trout Sheet

Preparation time: 5 minutes **Cooking time:** 20 minutes **Serves** 4
Ingredients:
- 3 tablespoons minced garlic, divided
- 2 tablespoons chili powder, divided

- 2 tablespoons olive oil, divided
- Sea salt
- 1 pound rainbow trout fillets
- 2 zucchini, sliced into rounds

Direction:
Preheat the oven to 425°F. Line a baking sheet with parchment paper. Mix 2 tablespoons of garlic, 1 tablespoon of chili powder, 1 tablespoon of olive oil, and a pinch of salt in a medium bowl. Generously coat both sides of the trout fillets with the garlic mixture and place them on one half of the baking sheet. Mix the remaining garlic, chili powder, olive oil, and another pinch of salt in another medium bowl. Add the zucchini to the bowl and stir to combine. Bake the fish for 20 minutes until slightly browned on the edges. Add the zucchini to the empty side of the baking sheet halfway through the cooking time. Enjoy immediately.
Nutrition: Calories: 186; Total fat: 9g; Saturated fat: 2g; Protein: 20g; Total carbohydrate: 6g; Fiber: 2g; Sodium: 158mg; Potassium: 724mg

Salmon Patties

Preparation time: 20 minutes **Cooking time:** 40 minutes **Serves** 4
Ingredients:
- ¼ cup quinoa, rinsed
- ½ cup water
- 2 (7½-ounce) cans of low-sodium deboned salmon, packed in water
- 1 tablespoon mustard
- 1 teaspoon Old Bay Seasoning
- 2 large eggs olive oil

Direction:
In a medium saucepan over high heat, combine the quinoa and water and bring to a boil. Reduce the heat to low, and simmer until the liquid is absorbed about 20 minutes. Remove from the heat, fluff with a fork, and let cool. Preheat the oven to 400°F. Line a baking sheet with parchment paper. Mix the salmon, mustard, and seasoning in a large bowl until well combined. Add the quinoa and eggs and blend well, then shape the mixture into 5 patties. Place the patties on the prepared baking sheet and bake for 20 minutes until they are slightly brown on the edges. Serve hot.
Nutrition: Calories: 202; Total fat: 10g; Saturated fat: 2g; Protein: 23g; Total carbohydrate: 6g; Fiber: 1g; Sodium: 480mg;

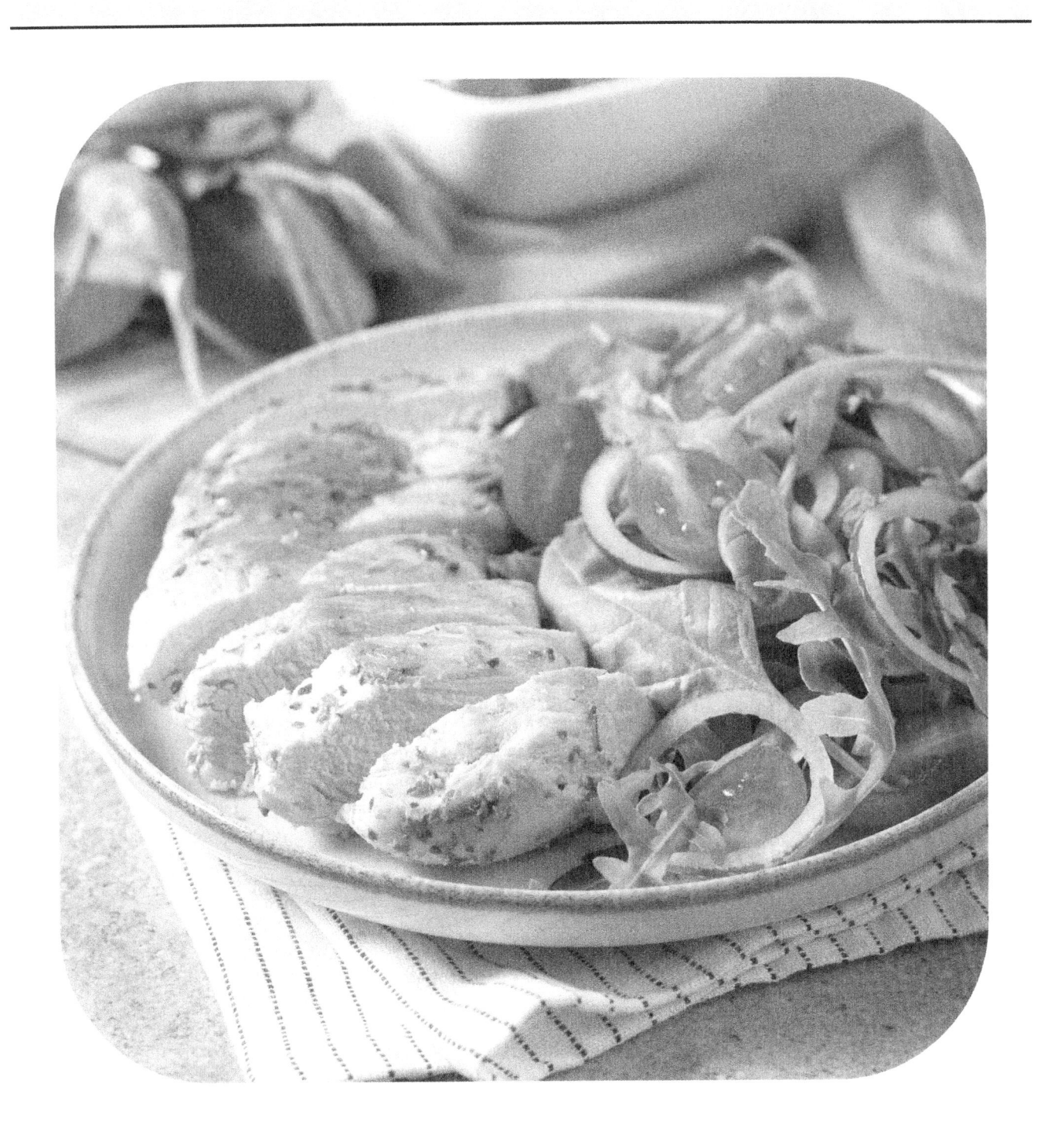

Chapter 10: POULTRY RECIPES

Garlicky Chicken Thighs with Vinegar

Preparation time: 10 minutes **Cooking time**: 20 minutes **Serves** 4
Ingredients:
- ¼ cup balsamic vinegar
- 2 tablespoons honey
- 1 tablespoon low-sodium soy sauce
- 3 cloves garlic, peeled and minced
- 1 tablespoon olive oil
- 1-pound boneless skinless chicken thighs
- ¼ teaspoon kosher or sea salt
- ¼ teaspoon ground black pepper

Direction:
Preheat the oven to 375°F. Whisk together the balsamic vinegar, honey, soy sauce, and garlic in a small bowl until combined. Heat the olive oil in an oven-safe skillet to medium-high. Season the chicken thighs with salt and black pepper. Once the pan is hot, place the chicken thighs into the pan and sear until crispy, about 5 minutes. Turn the chicken over and cook another 2 to 3 minutes. Add the sauce to the pan and bring to a simmer. Transfer to the oven and roast for 10 minutes until the internal temperature reaches 165°F. Serve immediately or place in microwaveable airtight containers and refrigerate for up to 5 days. To reheat, microwave on high for 1 to 2 minutes, until heated.
Nutrition: Calories: 227 | Fat: 10g | Protein: 21g | Carbohydrates: 12g| Fiber: 0g | Sugar: 9g| Sodium: 385mg

Zesty Chicken Kebabs with Eggplants

Preparation time: 10 minutes **Cooking time:** 15 minutes **Serves** 4
Ingredients:
- ½ cup plain nonfat Greek yogurt Zest and juice of 1 lemon
- 4 garlic cloves, peeled and minced
- 1-inch piece of fresh ginger, peeled and minced
- 2 tablespoons Garam Masala or store-bought garam masala
- ¼ teaspoon kosher or sea salt, divided
- ¼ teaspoon ground cayenne pepper
- 1 pound boneless skinless chicken breasts, cubed
- ½ eggplant, cubed
- 1-pint cherry tomatoes halved
- 1 tablespoon olive oil

Direction:
In a large zip-top plastic bag, combine the greek yogurt, lemon zest and juice, garlic, ginger, and garam masala with half of the salt and the cayenne pepper. Shake the bag with your hands to mix. Add the chicken cubes to the bag, seal, and place in the refrigerator for at least 30 minutes or overnight. Place the cubed eggplant and tomatoes in a small bowl, toss with the olive oil, and sprinkle with the remaining salt. Preheat the grill or grill pan over medium-high heat. Thread the marinated chicken, cubed eggplant, and tomatoes on skewers. Discard the extra marinade. Grill the kebabs for 15 to 18 minutes, turning regularly, until the chicken reaches 165°F, and the vegetables are soft and crispy.
Nutrition: Calories: 215 | Fat: 7g | Protein: 26g | Carbohydrates: 13g| Fiber: 3g | Sugar: 4g| Sodium: 522mg

Spaghetti with Chicken Meatballs

Preparation time: 10 minutes **Cooking time**: 30 minutes **Serves** 8
Ingredients:
- 2 pounds of ground chicken
- 2 large eggs
- ½ cup panko bread crumbs
- 1 tablespoon freshly grated Parmesan cheese
- 1 tablespoon Dijon mustard
- ½ tablespoon Italian seasoning
- ½ teaspoon kosher or sea salt
- ½ teaspoon ground black pepper
- ⅛ teaspoon crushed red pepper flakes
- 12 ounces whole-grain spaghetti
- 1 (24-ounce) jar of lower-sodium marinara sauce

Direction:
Preheat the oven to 375°F. Fit a baking sheet with a wire rack and coat it with cooking spray. Mix the ground chicken, eggs, bread crumbs, Parmesan cheese, Dijon mustard, Italian seasoning, salt, black pepper, and red pepper flakes in a mixing bowl. Form into 2-inch balls and line up on the wire rack. Bake for 18 to 22 minutes until the internal temperature reaches 165°F. While the meatballs cook, bring a large pot of water to a boil. Cook the spaghetti according to the package directions. Bring the marinara sauce to a simmer in a pot or a saucepan, stirring frequently. Serve the meatballs over the spaghetti and spoon the marinara sauce on top.
Nutrition: Calories: 426 | Fat: 15g | Protein: 29g |

Carbohydrates: 40g| Fiber: 5g | Sugar: 5g| Sodium: 394mg

Chicken Fajitas with Mango Salsa

Preparation time: 20 minutes **Cooking time:** 20 minutes **Serves** 4
Ingredients:
For the mango salsa:
- 1 mango, peeled, pitted, and diced
- ½ jalapeño, seeded and finely minced
- ¼ red onion, peeled and finely diced
- ½ cup fresh cilantro leaves, chopped
- Zest and juice of 2 limes
- ¼ teaspoon kosher or sea salt
- ¼ teaspoon ground black pepper

For the chicken fajitas:
- 1-pound boneless skinless chicken breasts, sliced into ½-inch strips
- ½ cup Chili Lime Marinade
- 2 red bell peppers, seeded and sliced
- 1 red onion, peeled and sliced
- 8 (6-inch) corn tortillas, toasted
- 1 avocado, peeled and sliced

Direction:
To make the mango salsa:
1. Combine the salsa ingredients in a bowl fitted with a lid and refrigerate until use.

To make the chicken fajitas:
Place the sliced chicken breast and marinade in a bowl fitted with a lid or in a large zip-top plastic bag and shake to coat. Refrigerate for at least 30 minutes. Heat a skillet over medium heat. Add the chicken and sauté for 3 to 4 minutes until opaque, then add the red bell pepper and onion and sauté for 3 to 4 more minutes, until the chicken is fully cooked and the bell peppers and onion are soft. Scoop the chicken, bell peppers, and onion mixture onto the corn tortillas and top with the avocado and mango salsa. For leftovers, store the chicken, bell pepper, and onion mixture in microwaveable airtight containers in the refrigerator for up to 5 days. Reheat the chicken in the microwave for 1 to 2 minutes, until heated through. Store the salsa in airtight containers in the refrigerator for up to 2 to 3 days.
Nutrition: Calories: 414 | Fat: 11g | Protein: 27g | Carbohydrates: 54g| Fiber: 6g | Sugar: 14g| Sodium: 458mg

Peppered Chicken Tortilla Casserole

Preparation time: 15 minutes **Cooking time:** 35 minutes **Serves** 8
Ingredients:
- 1 tablespoon olive oil
- 1 yellow onion, peeled and diced
- 1 red bell pepper, seeded and diced
- ½ jalapeño pepper, seeded and diced
- 2 pounds of ground chicken
- 4 cloves garlic, peeled and minced
- 2 tablespoons Taco Seasoning
- 8 (8-inch) whole-wheat flour tortillas
- 1 cup Enchilada Sauce or store-bought enchilada sauce
- ¾ cup shredded Mexican-style cheese
- 1 avocado, peeled and diced
- ¼ cup nonfat plain Greek yogurt
- ¼ cup fresh cilantro leaves, chopped

Direction:
Achieve a 375°F oven temperature. Apply cooking spray to a 9 by 9-inch baking pan. In a skillet over medium heat, warm the olive oil. Add the red bell pepper, onion, jalapenos, and sauté for 4 to 5 minutes, or until tender. When the chicken is done, add the ground chicken and continue to sauté for 5 to 7 minutes, regularly turning to break up the meat. The taco seasoning and garlic are combined. Take it off the heat. In the baking dish, arrange three tortillas in a line, overlapping as necessary, to cover the bottom. Place 1/3 of the meat, 1/3 of the sauce, and 1/3 of the cheese. Add two more layers, finishing with shredded cheese. The cheese should be melted and bubbled after 20 minutes in the oven.Slice into 8 wedges, then top with Greek yogurt, avocado, and cilantro. For up to five days, keep leftovers in microwaveable sealed containers. Heat up entirely in the microwave for 2 to 3 minutes.
Nutrition: Calories: 376 | Fat: 21g | Protein: 30g | Carbohydrates: 32g| Fiber: 5g | Sugar: 3g| Sodium: 535mg

White Chicken Chili

Preparation Time: 15 minutes **Cooking Time:** 20 minutes **Servings:** 1
Ingredients:
- 1 tbsp. extra-virgin olive oil
- 1 small yellow onion, diced
- 1 jalapeño, seeded and minced
- 2 cloves garlic, minced
- 1 tsp. dried oregano

- 1 tsp. ground cumin
- 2 (4.5 oz.) cans of green chilies
- 1 1/2 c. frozen corn
- 1/2 c. sour cream
- Freshly chopped cilantro for garnish
- 1/4 c. shredded Monterey Jack
- 1/4 c. crushed tortilla chips
- 3 boneless skinless chicken breasts, cut into thirds
- 5 c. low-sodium chicken broth
- Freshly ground black pepper
- Kosher salt
- 2 (15 oz.) cans of white beans

Directions:
Carefully warm the oil in a large saucepan over medium heat. It takes around 5 minutes to cook the onion and jalapeno until they are soft. Cook for approximately a minute, or until the cumin, oregano, and garlic are fragrant. Add the green chilies, chicken, and broth after seasoning with salt and pepper. For 10 to 12 minutes, or until the chicken is tender and cooked, bring to a boil, reduce heat to low, and cover. With two forks, shred the chicken and arrange it on a dish. Add the white beans and corn back to the stew and stir. Cook for 10 minutes at a simmer; mash about 1/4 of the beans with a wooden spoon. Carefully remove from heat and incorporate sour cream. Before serving, ladle chili into bowls and top with cilantro, cheese, and chips.
Nutrition: Calories: 351 | Fat: 20g | Protein: 26g | Carbohydrates: 0g| Fiber: 5g | Sugar: 3g | Sodium: 445mg

Parmesan Chicken Cutlets

Preparation Time: 15 minutes **Cooking Time:** 20 minutes **Servings:** 1
Ingredients:
- 4 boneless skinless chicken breasts
- Kosher salt
- Freshly ground black pepper
- 3 large eggs, beaten
- 2 tsp. lemon zest
- 1/2 tsp. cayenne pepper
- Vegetable oil
- Lemon wedges, for serving
- 1 c. all-purpose flour
- 2 1/4 c. panko
- 3/4 c. freshly grated Parmesan

Directions:
Cut the chicken breasts carefully in half crosswise with a sharp knife. Place the halves on a chopping board between two pieces of plastic wrap. Flatten the chicken to a thickness of 14" with a meat tenderizer or a rolling pin. Season appropriately on both sides of the chicken with salt and pepper. Separate the eggs and flour into two small basins. Combine panko, Parmesan, lemon zest, and cayenne in a third shallow dish. Season with salt and pepper to taste. I work one at a time, coating chicken cutlets in flour, eggs, and panko mixture. Two tablespoons oil, heated in a large pan over medium heat Cook until the chicken is brown and cooked through, 2 to 3 minutes per side. Working in batches as needed, add extra oil as needed. With lemon slices, serve.
Nutrition: Calories: 360 | Fat: 21g | Protein: 31g | Carbohydrates: 33g| Fiber: 5g | Sugar: 3g| Sodium: 516mg

Chicken Quesadillas

Preparation Time: 15 minutes **Cooking Time:** 20 minutes **Servings:** 1
Ingredients:
- 1 tbsp. extra-virgin olive oil
- 2 bell peppers, thinly sliced
- 1/2 tsp. chili powder
- 1/2 tsp. ground cumin
- 1/2 tsp. dried oregano
- 4 medium flour tortillas
- 2 c. shredded Monterey jack
- 2 c. shredded cheddar
- 1 ripe avocado, sliced
- 1 tbsp. vegetable oil
- 2 scallions, thinly sliced
- Sour cream, for serving
- 1/2 onion, thinly sliced
- Kosher salt
- Freshly ground black pepper
- 1 lb. boneless skinless chicken breasts, sliced into strips

Directions:
Warm the olive oil in a large pan over medium-high heat. Season the peppers and onion with salt and pepper. Cook for 5 minutes or until soft. Place on a platter. Over medium-high heat, heat the remaining tablespoon of vegetable oil. Season chicken with spices, salt, and pepper and cook, tossing periodically, for 8 minutes or until browned and cooked through. Place on a platter. The top half of a flour tortilla with a heavy dusting of both kinds of cheese, cooked chicken combination, pepper-onion mixture, a few slices of avocado, and green onions. Fold the second half of the tortilla and cook, flipping once, for 3 minutes per side, or until golden. Make four quesadillas in total. Cut into wedges and top it

with sour cream.
Nutrition: Calories: 346 | Fat: 23g | Protein: 29g | Carbohydrates: 31g| Fiber: 5g | Sugar: 3g| Sodium: 520 mg

Copycat Olive Garden Chicken Gnocchi Soup

Preparation Time: 15 minutes **Cooking Time:** 20 minutes **Servings:** 1
Ingredients:
- 2 tbsp. butter
- 1 (16 oz.) package gnocchi, fresh or thawed from frozen
- 1 medium onion, chopped
- 2 celery stalks, chopped
- 2 c. half and half
- 3 cloves garlic, minced
- 2 c. cooked chicken, shredded
- 2 c. baby spinach
- 1 medium carrot, julienned or shredded
- 6 c. low sodium or homemade chicken stock
- 3 sprigs thyme

Directions:
Melt butter in a large saucepan over medium-low heat. Cook until the onion, celery, and carrot are cooked for about 5 minutes. Cook for 30 to 1 minute, or until the garlic is aromatic. Deglaze with chicken stock (making sure to scrape the bottom of the pan to release any caramelized bits). Bring to a boil with the thyme sprigs. Reduce the heat to a gentle simmer and cook for 20 minutes to enable the flavors to emerge. Bring the liquid back to a boil after adding the half-and-half. Thyme sprigs should be removed and seasoned with salt and pepper to taste. Reduce the heat to medium-low and cook the gnocchi according to the package directions, or until just tender/firm. Cook until the spinach is slightly wilted. Spoon into serving dishes and serve.
Nutrition: Calories: 341 | Fat: 21g | Protein: 30g | Carbohydrates: 32g| Fiber: 5g | Sugar: 3g| Sodium: 522 mg

Lemon Pepper Chicken

Preparation Time: 15 minutes **Cooking Time:** 20 minutes **Servings:** 1
Ingredients:
- 1/2 c. all-purpose flour
- 1 tbsp. lemon-pepper seasoning
- 1 tsp. kosher salt
- 1/2 c. Chicken broth
- 2 tbsp. butter
- 2 cloves garlic, minced
- Freshly chopped parsley for garnish
- 2 lemons, divided
- 1 lb. boneless skinless chicken breasts halved
- 2 tbsp. extra-virgin olive oil

Directions:
Preheat the oven to 400°F. Combine flour, lemon pepper, salt, and one lemon zest in a medium mixing bowl. Toss the chicken breasts in the flour mixture until they are well covered. Cut the rest of the lemon into thin rounds. Heat the oil carefully in a large ovenproof skillet over medium-high heat. Cook until the bottom of the chicken is browned, about 5 minutes, then turn the chicken breasts. Add stock, butter, garlic, and lemon slices to the pan and bake until the chicken is cooked and the sauce is slightly reduced, about 5 minutes. Place the chicken on top of the sauce and decorate it with parsley. Combine flour, lemon pepper, salt, and one lemon zest in a medium mixing bowl. Toss the chicken breasts in the flour mixture until they are well covered. Cut the rest of the lemon into thin rounds. Heat the oil carefully in a large ovenproof skillet over medium-high heat. Cook until the bottom of the chicken is browned, about 5 minutes, then turn the chicken breasts. Add stock, butter, garlic, and lemon slices to the skillet and heat until the chicken is cooked and the sauce is slightly reduced, about 3 minutes. Place the chicken on top of the sauce and decorate it with parsley.
Nutrition: Calories: 323 | Fat: 21g | Protein: 30g | Carbohydrates: 32g| Fiber: 5g | Sugar: 3g| Sodium: 516 mg

Chapter 11: Vegetarian Main course Recipes

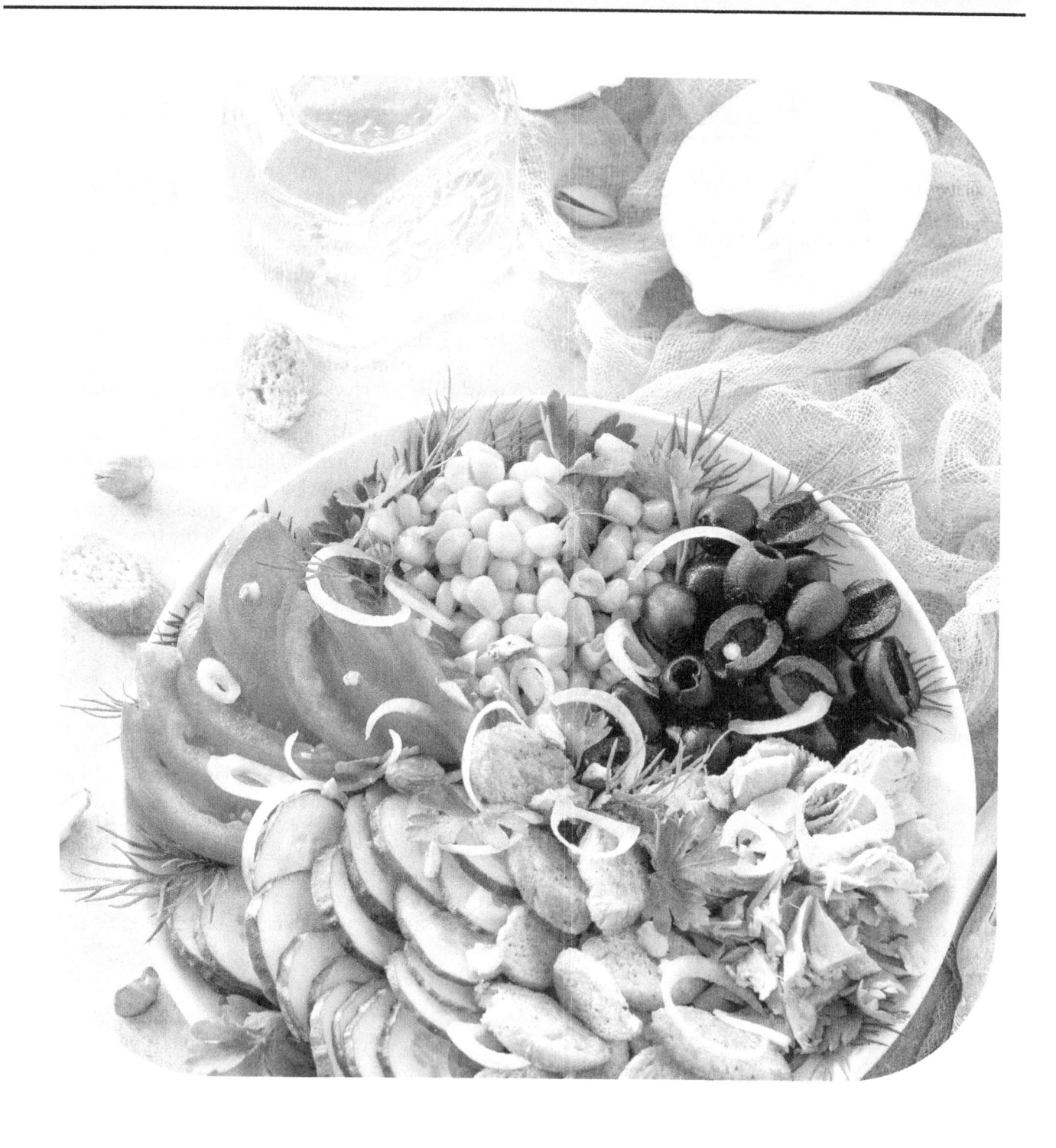

Zucchini with Cheesy Lasagna

Preparation time: 15 minutes **Cooking time:** 55 minutes **Serves** 10
Ingredients:
- 12 whole wheat lasagna noodles
- 1½ pounds cremini mushrooms, coarsely chopped
- 1 medium zucchini, cut into ½-inch pieces
- 1 medium yellow squash, cut into ½-inch pieces
- 2 tablespoons extra-virgin olive oil
- 1 large onion, chopped
- 4 garlic cloves, minced
- 3 cups spinach leaves
- 1 cup no-salt-added tomato sauce
- 1 (6-ounce) can of no-salt-added tomato paste
- 1 (28-ounce) can of no-salt-added crushed tomatoes
- ½ teaspoon salt
- 1 teaspoon freshly ground black pepper
- 3 large eggs, beaten
- 1 (15-ounce) container 1% cottage cheese
- 4 cups shredded part-skim low-moisture mozzarella cheese, divided
- ¾ cup grated Parmesan cheese, divided
- 1 tablespoon dried basil
- 1 teaspoon garlic powder
- 1 teaspoon onion powder

Direction:
Preheat the oven to 350°F. Bring a large pot of water to a boil. Add the lasagna noodles and cook until al dente according to the package directions. Drain and lay them flat on a sheet of aluminum foil. In a large sauté pan or deep skillet, dry-sauté the mushrooms over medium heat until moisture releases. Then add the zucchini and squash. When the mushrooms are no longer releasing moisture, add the oil, onion, garlic, and spinach. Sauté, stirring, for 2 to 3 minutes, or until all the vegetables have softened. Add the tomato sauce, paste, and crushed tomatoes, and stir in the salt and pepper. Mix the eggs, cottage cheese, 2½ cups of mozzarella cheese, ½ cup of Parmesan cheese, basil, garlic powder, and onion powder in a large bowl. In a 9-by-13-inch baking dish, spread some tomato and vegetable sauce mixture to cover the bottom. Make 3 layers, Top with a final layer of noodles, the remaining 1½ cups of mozzarella, and ¼ cup of Parmesan cheeses. Cover with foil and bake for 40 minutes. Remove the foil and bake for 10 to 15 minutes, or until browned and bubbling. Let cool completely before cutting into 10 portions. Place a portion in each of 10 containers.
Nutrition: Calories: 438 | Fat: 17g | Protein: 28g | Carbohydrates: 44g| Fiber: 8g | Sugar: 5g| Sodium: 782mg

Celery with Mushroom Bolognese

Preparation time: 10 minutes **Cooking time:** 25 minutes **Serves** 4
Ingredients:
- 8 ounces whole wheat penne pasta
- 2 tablespoons extra-virgin olive oil
- 1 small onion, diced
- 1 large carrot, diced
- 2 celery stalks, diced
- 4 garlic cloves, minced
- 1-pound mushrooms, diced
- ⅔ cup dry red wine
- 1 bay leaf
- 2 cups low-sodium vegetable broth
- 1 (15-ounce) can of no-salt-added tomato sauce
- 1 teaspoon Italian seasoning
- ¼ teaspoon freshly ground black pepper
- ¼ teaspoon red pepper flakes (optional)
- ½ cup grated Parmesan cheese

Direction:
Bring a large pot of water to a boil. Add the pasta and cook until al dente according to the package directions. Drain well. Meanwhile, heat the oil over medium-high heat in a large sauté pan or deep skillet. Add the onion, carrot, and celery and cook for 5 to 7 minutes, until the vegetables are soft and the onion is translucent. Add the garlic and mushrooms and cook for 4 to 5 minutes, or until the mushrooms are browned. Stir in the wine, add the bay leaf, bring to a boil, and cook for 2 to 3 minutes, or until the wine is reduced by half. Remove the bay leaf. Add the vegetable broth, tomato sauce, Italian seasoning, black pepper, and red pepper flakes (if using). In a large bowl, toss the drained pasta with the sauce. Divide into 4 storage containers and top each serving with 2 tablespoons of Parmesan cheese.
Nutrition: Calories: 456 | Fat: 12g | Protein: 18g | Carbohydrates: 70g| Fiber: 10g | Sugar: 5g| Sodium: 344mg

Chili Bean Mix with Scallion

Preparation time: 10 minutes **Cooking time:** 30 minutes **Serves** 6
Ingredients:
- 2 tablespoons extra-virgin olive oil
- 1 medium onion, diced

- 1 green bell pepper, diced
- 2 garlic cloves, minced
- 1 (28-ounce) can of no-salt-added crushed tomatoes
- 1 tablespoon chili powder
- 1 teaspoon ground cumin
- 1 (15-ounce) can of no-salt-added black beans, drained and rinsed
- 1 (15-ounce) can of no-salt-added pinto beans, drained and rinsed
- 1 (15-ounce) can of no-salt-added kidney beans, drained and rinsed
- 1 (15-ounce) can of no-salt-added navy beans, drained and rinsed
- 1 (15-ounce) can of no-salt-added chickpeas, drained and rinsed
- 10 scallions, chopped

Direction:
In a large pot, heat the oil over medium-high heat. Add the onion and bell pepper and cook for 5 to 7 minutes until the onion is translucent. Add the garlic and cook for 1 minute. Stir in the crushed tomatoes, chili powder, cumin, black beans, pinto beans, kidney beans, navy beans, and chickpeas. Reduce the heat to a simmer and cook, frequently stirring, for 20 minutes to thicken slightly and blend the flavors. Divide among 6 storage containers. Store the scallions separately. Top the chili with the scallions after reheating to serve.
Nutrition: Calories: 425 | Fat: 7g | Protein: 23g | Carbohydrates: 67g| Fiber: 23g | Sugar: 8g| Sodium: 58mg

Cheese crepes with spinach

Preparation time: 10 minutes **Cooking time:** 20 minutes **Serves** 8
Ingredients:
- Nonstick cooking spray
- 1 cup whole wheat flour
- 2 large eggs
- ½ cup 1% milk
- ½ cup water
- ¼ teaspoon salt
- 2 teaspoons extra-virgin olive oil, divided
- 1 garlic clove, minced
- 1 cup chopped spinach
- 1 cup chopped kale leaves
- 1 cup chopped fresh parsley
- 1 tablespoon fresh thyme
- ¼ teaspoon freshly ground black pepper
- ¼ cup shredded part-skim low-moisture mozzarella cheese

Direction:
Preheat the broiler to 500°F. Coat a 9-by-13-inch broiler-safe baking dish with cooking spray. In a large bowl, whisk together the flour and eggs. Gradually add the milk, water, and salt, stirring until well combined. Grease a nonstick skillet with 1 teaspoon of oil and heat over medium-high heat. Pour ¼ cup of the batter into the skillet. Tilt the skillet in a circular motion, so the batter coats the surface evenly. Cook the crêpe for about 2 minutes, or until the bottom is lightly browned. Repeat to make a total of 8 crêpes. Heat the remaining 1 teaspoon of oil in a separate skillet over medium heat. Add the garlic and cook, stirring rapidly, for 30 seconds. Add the spinach, kale, parsley, thyme, and pepper. Cook for 3 to 5 minutes, occasionally stirring, or until the spinach and kale have wilted. Divide the spinach mixture and mozzarella cheese evenly among the crêpes. Roll up the crêpes and place them in the prepared baking dish. Set under the broiler for a few minutes, just to melt the cheese, keeping a close eye on it. Divide the crêpes among 4 storage containers.
Nutrition: Calories: 253 | Fat: 15g | Protein: 11g | Carbohydrates: 26g| Fiber: 4g | Sugar: 8g| Sodium: 255mg

Creamy Vegetable Quiche

Preparation time: 10 minutes **Cooking time:** 55 minutes **Serves** 8
Ingredients:
- 1 (9-inch) unbaked deep-dish piecrust
- 1 tablespoon extra-virgin olive oil
- ½ medium red onion, finely chopped
- 1 large green bell pepper, chopped
- ½ cup sliced cremini mushrooms
- 1 small zucchini, chopped
- 1 large tomato, chopped
- 6 large eggs
- ½ cup 1% milk
- 2 tablespoons all-purpose flour
- 2 teaspoons dried basil
- ½ teaspoon salt
- ½ teaspoon freshly ground black pepper
- 1½ cups shredded Monterey Jack cheese, divided

Direction:
Preheat the oven to 350°F. Bake the crust for 7 to 8 minutes to set. Remove from the oven, but leave the range on. In a large skillet, heat the oil over medium heat. Add the onion and sauté for about 1 minute. Add the bell pepper, mushrooms, zucchini, and tomato and cook for 5 to 7 minutes, or until soft. Remove from the heat and set aside. Whisk together

the eggs, milk, flour, basil, salt, and black pepper in a medium bowl. Stir in 1 cup of Monterey Jack cheese. Pour the mixture into the baked pie crust. Top with the remaining ½ cup of cheese. Bake for 40 to 50 minutes or until the mixture is cooked through. Cool for 10 minutes before cutting into 8 wedges. Divide the wedges among 8 storage containers.
Nutrition: Calories: 266 | Fat: 17g | Protein: 12g | Carbohydrates: 17g| Fiber: 1g | Sugar: 7g| Sodium: 422mg

Cannellini Bean Pizza

Preparation time: 10 minutes **Cooking time:** 15 minutes **Serves:** 3
Ingredients:
- Aluminum foil
- 1½ cups canned cannellini beans drained and rinsed
- ½ cup whole-wheat flour
- 2 large whole eggs
- 1 tbsp nutritional yeast
- 4 tbsp low-sodium tomato puree
- ½ cup entire white mushrooms, thinly sliced
- ½ cup reduced fat cheese blend, shredded
- 1 tbsp garlic, minced
- 1 tsp garlic powder

Directions:
Warm the oven to 450°F, gas mark 8. Line a baking sheet with aluminum foil. Combine the cannellini beans, whole-wheat flour, whole eggs, and nutritional yeast in a food processor or blender. Process for 1 minute until it forms a doughy consistency. Place the bean mixture on the baking sheet, and spread evenly. The combination will not be like pizza dough but slightly sticky. Use a spatula to spread evenly. Bake for 10 minutes, until the edges are lightly browned. Remove the base from the oven, and spread the tomato puree, sliced mushrooms, cheese blend, minced garlic, and garlic powder evenly over the pizza. Bake for 5 minutes, until the cheese, has melted. Cut into 8 slices and serve warm.
Nutrition: Calories: 290, Total Fat: 9g, Saturated Fat: 3g, Cholesterol: 21mg, Sodium: 206mg, Total Carbs: 36g, Net Carbs: 2.8g, Fiber: 8g, Protein: 19g

Garbanzo Bean Curry

Preparation time: 10 minutes **Cooking time:** 30 minutes **Serves:** 4
Ingredients:
- 1 tbsp olive oil
- 1 small onion, finely chopped
- 2 cups stir-fry vegetables, fresh or frozen
- 1 tbsp ginger, grated
- 2 tsp mild curry paste
- 1 tsp ground turmeric
- 1 (14 oz) can dice no-salt-added tomatoes with their juices
- 1 (15 oz) can of garbanzo beans, rinsed and drained
- ¼ cup almond butter
- 2 cups reduced-sodium vegetable stock

Directions:
Heat the olive oil over medium-high heat in a large, heavy-bottom pan. Add the chopped onion, and cook for 4 to 5 minutes, until translucent. Add the stir-fry vegetables, and cook for 3 to 4 minutes. Add the grated ginger, mild curry paste, and ground turmeric, cook for 1 minute, and mix to combine. Stir in the diced tomatoes with their juice, garbanzo beans, almond butter, and vegetable stock, and allow to boil. Allow simmering on low, occasionally stirring, for 5 to 10 minutes, until warmed. Serve hot.
Nutrition: Calories: 308; Total Fat: 14g; Saturated Fat: 1g; Cholesterol: 0mg; Sodium: 348mg; Total Carbs: 34g; Fiber: 10g; Protein: 12g

Pinto Bean Tortilla

Preparation time: 10 minutes **Cooking time:** 5 minutes **Serves:** 4
Ingredients:
- 1 (15 oz) can of no-salt-added pinto beans, rinsed and drained
- ¼ cup fresh tomato salsa
- ¾ cup reduced fat cheese blend, divided
- 1 medium green bell pepper, seeded and chopped, divided
- 2 tbsp olive oil, divided
- 4 large, whole-grain tortillas

Directions:
In a food processor, blend the pinto beans and tomato salsa. Alternatively, mash them in a large mixing bowl with a fork or a potato masher. Spread ½ cup of the bean mixture on each tortilla. Sprinkle each tortilla with 3 tbsp cheese blend and ¼ cup of chopped green bell pepper. Fold in half. Heat a large, heavy bottom pan over medium heat. Add 1 tbsp of olive oil to the pan. Place the first two folded tortillas in the pan. Cover, and cook for 2 minutes until the tortillas are crispy on the bottom. Flip, and cook for 2 minutes until crispy on the other side. Use 1 tbsp of olive oil for cooking the remaining two tortillas.
Nutrition: Calories: 438; Total Fat: 21g; Saturated Fat: 5g; Cholesterol: 21mg; Sodium: 561mg; Total Carbs: 46g; Fiber: 12g; Protein: 17g

Green frittata

Preparation Time: 15 minutes **Cooking Time:** 20 minutes **Servings:** 1
Ingredients:
- 1 cup basil leaves
- 1 cup flat-leaf parsley leaves
- 1½ cups baby kale, plus extra leaves to serve
- 1 zucchini, shaved in strips
- 4 stalks of asparagus
- Lemon juice to serve
- 2 cups baby spinach
- 6 eggs
- 1 lb ricotta
- ¼ cup (20g) parmesan
- 2 tbsp extra virgin olive oil, plus extra to serve
- 1 onion, sliced
- 2 garlic cloves, crushed

Directions:
Heat the oven to 180°C. Combine the herbs and spinach in a food processor and pulse until finely chopped. Whiz the eggs, ricotta, parmesan, and seasoning until smooth. In a frying pan, carefully heat the oil over medium heat. Cook for 2-3 minutes, or until the onion is softened, then add the garlic and cook for 1 minute, or until fragrant. Combine the young kale and zucchini strips in a mixing bowl. Take the pan off the heat. Stir in the egg mixture to incorporate and distribute the ingredients evenly in the pan. Cook for 20-25 minutes until puffed and golden on top. Remove from the oven and leave aside for 5 minutes before sliding out of the pan. Serve with asparagus, other kale leaves, and a sprinkle of lemon juice and olive oil.
Nutrition: Calories: 273 | Fat: 16g | Protein: 11g | Carbohydrates: 26g| Fiber: 4g | Sugar: 8g| Sodium: 271mg

Lemon Chicken Orzo Soup

Preparation time: 10 minutes **Cooking time:** 20 minutes **Servings:** 6
Ingredients:
- 2 tbsp. olive oil
- 2 tbsp. parsley leaves
- 1 lb. boneless chicken
- 1 lemon juice
- Kosher salt
- Black pepper
- 1 spring rosemary
- 3 cloves garlic
- ¾ cup orzo pasta
- ½ tsp. dried thyme
- 1 onion
- 2 bay leaves
- 3 carrots
- 5 cups chicken stocks
- 2 stalks celery

Directions:
Pour olive oil stockpot over medium heat. Rub boneless chicken with black pepper and salt. Add the rubbed chicken to the stockpot. Cook it for 2 to 3 minutes until it becomes golden. Again, heat the oil in the stockpot and cook celery, carrots, and onion, stirring for 3 to 4 minutes until soft. Add the thyme and blend it until fragrant. Add the water, chicken stock, and bay leaves, mix well, and boil. Then, add the chicken, orzo, and rosemary until soft for 12 minutes and stirring constantly. Add the parsley and lemon juice and mix well. Sprinkle salt and pepper on it. Serve and enjoy.
Nutrition: Calories: 167 kcal | Fat: 4.1 g | Protein: 12.1 g | Carbs: 21.7 g | 12 mg Sodium

Spiced eggplant fritters

Preparation Time: 15 minutes **Cooking Time:** 20 minutes **Servings:** 1
Ingredients:
- 2 eggplants, cut into 1cm-thick rounds
- 1/2 cup (75g) plain flour, seasoned
- 1 tsp ground sumac
- 2 eggs
- 2 cups (100g) panko breadcrumbs
- 2 spring onions, thinly sliced
- 1 cup red vein sorrel, to serve
- Olive oil, to shallow fry
- 1 cup (280g) thick Greek-style yogurt
- Juice of 1 lemon
- 1 garlic clove, crushed
- 4 heirloom tomatoes, sliced
- Seeds of 1 pomegranate

Directions:
Sprinkle 2 tsp sea salt flakes over the eggplant in a colander placed over a basin. Allow for a 30-minute rest to remove any bitterness. Rinse with cold water and wipe dry with a paper towel. In a mixing dish, combine the flour and sumac. In a separate container, softly whisk the eggs. In a third bowl, combine the panko. Dip eggplant in flour, then in egg, let excess drop off, and last in panko. In a large nonstick frypan, heat 5mm oil over medium heat. Cook eggplant in batches for 5-6 minutes on each side until brown and soft. Maintain your body temperature. Rep with the leftover eggplant. Combine the yogurt, lemon juice, and garlic in a mixing dish. Season. Top with patties, tomato,

pomegranate seeds, spring onion, and sorrel on a serving platter. Serve right away.
Nutrition: Calories: 201 kcal | Fat: 5.1 g | Protein: 13.1 g | Carbs: 21.9 g | 14 mg Sodium

Broccoli Rice Casserole

Preparation time: 10 minutes **Cooking Time:** 60 minutes **Servings:** 6
Ingredients:
- 1 1/2 cups wild rice
- 6 cups broccoli
- 2 cups reduced-sodium cream of mushroom soup
- 2 cups low-fat cheddar cheese, shredded

Instructions
Preheat the oven to 325°F before starting. Prepare wild rice as directed on the package. Layer rice in the bottom of a 9 × 9-inch (23 x 23-cm) casserole pan. Broccoli should be steamed for 5 minutes before being layered on top of rice. Toss the soup with the cheese and distribute it on top of the broccoli. Bake for 45 minutes, uncovered.
Nutrition: Calories: 293 kcal, protein: 20 g, carbohydrates: 44 g, Fat: 5 g, Cholesterol:12 mg, Fiber: 5 g

Grilled Eggplant and Tomato Pasta

Preparation time: 5 minutes **Cooking Time:** 25 minutes **Servings:** 4
Ingredients:
- 2 teaspoons of chopped fresh oregano.
- 4 tablespoons of olive oil; extra-virgin, divided.
- 1 pound of chopped plum tomatoes,
- ½ teaspoon of ground pepper
- 1 grated clove of garlic,
- ½ teaspoon of salt
- ¼ teaspoon of crushed red pepper
- ½ cup of chopped fresh basil.
- 1 ½ pound of eggplant,
- 1/2-inch-thick slices
- ¼ cup of crumbled feta cheese or shaved Ricotta Salata
- 8 ounces of whole-wheat penne

Direction:
Bring a big saucepan of water to a boil. Preheat the grill to medium-high heat. In a large mixing bowl, combine 3 tablespoons of oil, crushed red pepper, tomatoes, garlic, pepper, oregano, and salt. Brush the remaining one tablespoon of oil over the eggplant. Grill for 4 minutes on each side, flipping once until cooked and browned in places. Allow 10 minutes for cooling. Chop them into bite-size pieces and add to the tomatoes with basil. In the meanwhile, prepare the pasta according to the package instructions. Drain. Toss the tomato mixture with the spaghetti and serve. Cheese should be sprinkled on top.
Nutrition: Calories: 449 kcal, protein: 13.5 g, carbohydrates: 62.1 g, Fat: 19.2 g, Cholesterol: 8.3 mg, Fiber: 3 g

Potato and Vegetable Casserole

Preparation time: 10 minutes **Cooking Time:** 30 minutes **Servings:** 6
Ingredients:
- 6 potatoes
- 2 tablespoons olive oil
- 1 cup onion, sliced
- 2 cups cabbage, chopped
- 2 cups cauliflower, chopped
- 1 teaspoon garlic, crushed
- 1 cup plain fat-free yogurt
- 2 cups canned white kidney beans
- 1/4 cup fresh dill, chopped
- 1/2 teaspoon paprika

Direction:
Preheat the oven to 325°F. Boil or microwave the potatoes until nearly done. When cool enough, peel if desired. Heat the olive oil in a large skillet over medium-high heat. Sauté the onions until soft. Add the cabbage, cauliflower, and garlic, and fry until the cabbage and cauliflower are tender. Add the yogurt to the vegetable mixture. Drain and rinse the white beans and add them to the vegetable mixture. Mix thoroughly and set aside. Slice the potatoes into rounds and put half the slices on the bottom of a 9 x 13-inch (23 x 33-cm) baking dish sprayed with nonstick vegetable oil. Spread the vegetable mixture over the potatoes. Cover with the remaining potatoes. Sprinkle with dill and paprika. Bake for 20 minutes.
Nutrition: Calories: 462 kcal, protein: 17 g, carbohydrates: 88 g, Fat: 6 g, Cholesterol: 1 mg, Fiber: 12 g

Cereal bowl with cashew and tahini sauce

Preparation time: 20 minutes **Cooking Time:** 0 minutes **Servings:** 1
Ingredients:
- ¼ cup of packed parsley leaves
- ½ cup of water

- ¼ teaspoon of salt
- 1 tablespoon of cider vinegar or lemon juice
- ½ teaspoon of tamari or soy sauce; extra-virgin
- ¾ cup of unsalted cashews
- ½ cup of cooked lentils
- 1 tablespoon of olive oil; extra-virgin
- ¼ cup of grated raw beet
- ½ cup of cooked quinoa
- ¼ cup of chopped bell pepper
- ½ cup of shredded red cabbage
- ¼ cup of grated carrot

For garnish,
- 1 tablespoon of chopped Toasted cashews.
- ¼ cup of sliced cucumber

Direction:
Mix water, tamari (soy sauce), cashews, lemon juice (or vinegar), oil, parsley, and salt in a blender. In the middle of a shallow serving dish, combine lentils and quinoa. Cabbage, carrot, beet, pepper, and cucumber go on top. Two tablespoons of cashew sauce are spooned over the top (save the extra sauce for another use). If desired, garnish with cashews.
Nutrition: Calories: 361 kcal, protein: 16.6 g, carbohydrates: 53.9 g, Fat: 10.1 g, Cholesterol: 1 mg, Fiber: 6 g

Creamy Zucchini And Potato Soup

Preparation Time: 15 minutes **Cooking Time:** 20 minutes **Servings:** 1
Ingredients:
- 2 tablespoons extra virgin olive oil
- 2 large zucchinis, cut into 1-inch cubes
- 2 large russet potatoes, cut into 1-inch cubes
- 4 cups vegetable broth
- 1 tablespoon lemon juice
- 1 tablespoon curry powder
- ½ cup chopped onion, about ½ medium onion
- ½ cup diced celery, about two stalks
- 1 clove garlic
- Salt & pepper to taste

Directions:
Warm the olive oil in a large saucepan over medium heat. Cook for approximately 5 minutes or until the onion and celery are tender and transparent. Cook for another 2 minutes after adding the garlic. Cook for about 5 minutes or until the zucchini begins to caramelize. Combine the potatoes and the vegetable broth in a mixing bowl. Bring to a boil, reduce to low heat, cover, and cook for 15 minutes, or until the potatoes are fork tender. If you're using an immersion blender, puree the soup until it's creamy. If using a regular blender, add the soup to the blender in stages and process until smooth, back to the pot. Season with salt and pepper, and stir in the lemon juice and curry powder. Seasoning should be tasted and adjusted as needed. Garnish with a drizzle of olive oil, torn parsley, and cracked black pepper, and serve hot.
Nutrition: Calories: 350 kcal, protein: 14.6 g, carbohydrates: 61.9 g, Fat: 10.1 g, Cholesterol: 1 mg, Fiber: 5 g

Vegan Ratatouille

Preparation Time: 15 minutes **Cooking Time:** 20 minutes **Servings:** 1
Ingredients:
- 1 tablespoon olive oil
- 1 large onion, diced
- 4 cloves garlic, chopped finely
- 1 large eggplant/aubergine, diced into ¾-inch pieces
- 2 large zucchinis, diced into ¾-inch pieces
- 2 large bell peppers were deseeded & cut into ¾-inch pieces
- 6 cups of about eight large fresh tomatoes, chopped into chunky pieces
- 1 teaspoon fennel seed, optional but recommended
- 1 teaspoon freshly ground black pepper
- 2 teaspoons salt
- 1 teaspoon dried rosemary or one fresh sprig, or one teaspoon herbs, de Provence
- 1 large bay leaf

Directions:
Heat the olive oil in a big skillet that holds at least 5 to 6 quarts/liters over medium heat. Feel free to increase the amount of olive oil if desired; O) (If you wish to keep the recipe oil-free, sauté with a bit of water instead.) When the oil is heated, add the onions and fry for 7 to 8 minutes or until they are transparent. Cook for another 2 minutes, constantly stirring, after adding the garlic. Add the remaining ingredients, give it a thorough mix, and bring it to a steady boil. Cook for 15 to 20 minutes, occasionally stirring, or until the vegetables are soft and the tomatoes have mostly broken down. Before serving, remove the bay leaf.
Nutrition: Calories: 323 kcal, protein: 15.6 g, carbohydrates: 49.9 g, Fat: 11.1 g, Cholesterol: 1 mg, Fiber: 6 g

Homemade Rice Pilaf

Preparation Time: 15 minutes **Cooking Time:** 20

minutes **Servings:** 1
Ingredients:
- 2 tablespoons olive oil
- 1/2 large onion
- 3 large garlic cloves, minced
- 1/2 cup orzo
- 1 cup long-grain white rice rinsed
- 3 cups stock
- 1/4 teaspoon coriander
- 1/4 teaspoon garlic powder
- 1/4 teaspoon onion powder
- 1/4 teaspoon paprika
- 1/4 teaspoon salt
- 1/2 cup fresh parsley, chopped

Directions:
Heat one tablespoon of olive oil over medium heat in a cast-iron pan, deep skillet, or pot. Sauté the garlic and onion for 60-90 seconds. If you're using frozen stock, remove it from the freezer and let it come to room temperature. Alternatively, you may cook it in a saucepan or microwave it in a Pyrex measuring cup Stir in the orzo well to coat it. 3 minutes, stirring often. Add the remaining one tablespoon of olive oil, followed by the rice. To ensure that all rice is covered in the oil, give it a good stir. Toast rice for 4-5 minutes or until transparent. Stir in the spices, garlic powder, onion powder, coriander, paprika, and salt to the rice. Slowly pour in the heated or room temperature stock. Turn the heat up to high, bring it to a boil, then reduce it to medium/low (a gentle simmer), cover, and leave to cool for 15 minutes (or follow the cooking time on your rice package). Remove the lid only after the cooking time is up! After 15 minutes, take rice from heat and set it aside for 3 minutes, covered. Remove the cover, decorate with parsley, and fluff with a fork before serving.
Nutrition: Calories: 343 kcal, protein: 16.9 g, carbohydrates: 51.6 g, Fat: 10.8 g, Cholesterol: 1 mg, Fiber: 7 g

Fried Rice Tom Yum

Preparation Time: 15 minutes **Cooking Time:** 20 minutes **Servings:** 1
Ingredients:
- 3 cloves garlic minced
- 2 kaffir lime leaves roughly chopped
- 2 Thai red chili sliced
- 1 tablespoon tom yum paste
- 1 medium carrot diced
- 2 cups cooked brown/white rice (refrigerated overnight)
- ½ cup frozen green peas
- 1 tablespoon soy sauce or tamari
- 1 stalk of green onion chopped
- lime juice to serve

Directions:
Heat a tablespoon of oil in a cast-iron skillet or nonstick pan over medium-high heat. Begin by sautéing the garlic, chili, and kaffir lime leaves for about 1-2 minutes or until aromatic. Three garlic cloves, 2 Thai red chilies, and two kaffir lime leaves. Cook for another minute, stirring regularly, after adding the tom yum paste. 1 tbsp. Tom yum paste. After that, add the carrot. Cook for 3-4 minutes, stirring regularly until softened. One carrot, medium. Now stir in the rice, peas, and soy sauce. Cook for another 2-3 minutes, or until everything is well heated. Taste it and add additional soy sauce if necessary. 12 cups frozen green peas, 2 cups cooked brown/white rice, and one tablespoon soy sauce Stir in the green onions, squeeze in the lime juice, and serve!
Nutrition: Calories: 290 kcal, protein: 13.6 g, carbohydrates: 42.9 g, Fat: 8.1 g, Cholesterol: 1 mg, Fiber: 5 g

Healthy banana cookies with oatmeal

Preparation Time: 15 minutes **Cooking Time:** 20 minutes **Servings:** 1
Ingredients:
- 2 ripe bananas
- 1 cup rolled oats (oatmeal or porridge oats work well)
- Optional: One small handful of sesame seeds (toasted)
- 1 tsp cinnamon
- 1 small handful of raisins
- 1 small handful of walnuts (crumbled)

Directions:
Preheat the oven to 360°F. Mash the bananas in a bowl until they're mushy. Two bananas, ripe. Combine the cup of oats with any of the optional ingredients. 1 cup rolled oats, one teaspoon cinnamon, a small handful of raisins, a small handful of walnuts, and a tiny handful of sesame seeds. Stir until everything is well combined. Place baking paper on the tray to prevent the cookies from sticking. If you don't have any, grease the baking sheet with butter (or olive oil if you're vegan). Form the cookie shape, take a spoon and scoop a good amount of the batter onto the baking tray, as shown in the photo above. It's pretty quick and straightforward. It is placed in the oven for around 15 - 20 minutes.

Nutrition: Calories: 292 kcal, protein: 15.1 g, carbohydrates: 50.6 g, Fat: 9.4 g, Cholesterol: 1 mg, Fiber: 5 g

Chapter 12: SNACK RECIPES

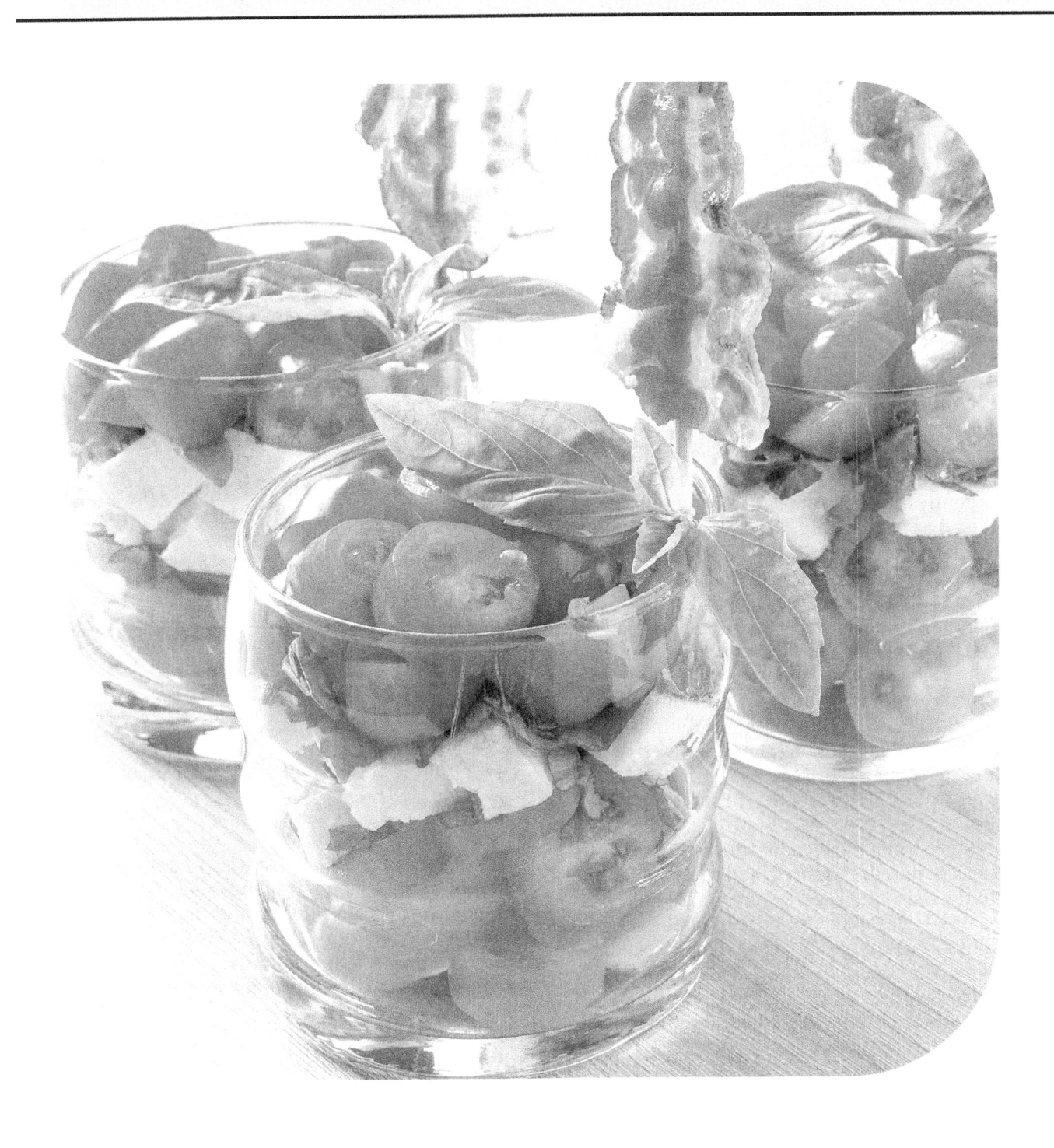

Hummus

Preparation time: 25 minutes **Cooking time:** 20 minutes plus chilling **Serves** 1
Ingredients:
- can (15 ounces) garbanzo beans/chickpeas: rinsed & drained
- 1/4 cup of fresh lemon juice
- 1/2 cup of tahini
- 1/2 teaspoon of baking soda
- 1/2 teaspoon of kosher salt
- 1 tablespoon of minced garlic
- 1/4 cup of cold water
- 1/2 teaspoon of ground cumin
- 1 tablespoon of extra virgin olive oil

Optional:
roasted garbanzo beans, Olive oil, ground sumac, toasted sesame seeds,
Direction:
Place the garbanzo beans and enough water to cover them by 1 inch in a large saucepan. Rub the beans together gently to release the outer skin. Pour off the water as well as any floating skins. Drain 2-3 times after repeating steps unless no skins float to the top. Return to saucepan; stir in baking soda and 1 inch of water. Bring to a boil, then turn off the heat. Cook for 20-25 minutes, or until beans are soft and begin to come apart. Meanwhile, puree the garlic, lemon juice, and salt in a blender until smooth. Allow 10 minutes to stand before straining and discarding the solids. Cumin is added at this point. Combine tahini and olive oil in a small bowl. Blend the beans with the cold water in a blender. Cover loosely with cover and process until absolutely smooth. Stir in the lemon mixture in the food processor. Slowly drizzle in the tahini mixture while the blender runs, scraping down the sides as required. If desired, add more salt and cumin to the seasoning. Refrigerate for at least 30 minutes after transferring the mixture to the serving bowl. Additional toppings or olive oil may be added if desired.
Nutrition: Calories: 250 kcal, Protein: 7 g, Carbohydrates: 15 g, Fat: 19 g, Cholesterol: 0 mg, Fiber: 5 g

Honey-Lime Berry Salad

Preparation time: 15 minutes **Cooking time:** 0 minutes **Serves** 10
Ingredients:
- Granny Smith apples, cubed
- 1/4 cup honey
- 4 cups fresh strawberries, halved cups fresh blueberries medium
- 1/3 cup lime juice
- 2 tablespoons minced fresh mint

Direction:
Combine strawberries, blueberries, and apples in a large mixing dish. Combine the lime juice, honey, and mint in a small mixing bowl. Toss the fruit in the dressing to coat. Per Serving Calories: 93 kcal, Protein: 1 g, Carbohydrates: 24 g, Fat: 0 g, Cholesterol: 0 mg, Fiber: 3 g Smoky Cauliflower Prep time:30 minutes| Cook time:0 minutes| Serves 8 1 tablespoons of olive oil 1 large head cauliflower: 1-inch florets: about 9 cups 3/4 teaspoon of salt 1 teaspoon of smoked paprika tablespoons of minced fresh parsley 2 garlic cloves: minced In a large mixing bowl, place the cauliflower. Combine the oil, paprika, and salt. Drizzle the dressing over the cauliflower and toss to coat. Fill a 15x10x1-inch baking pan halfway with the batter. Bake for 10 minutes at 450°F, uncovered. Add the garlic and mix well. Bake for 10-15 minutes, stirring periodically until cauliflower is soft and lightly browned. Serve with a parsley garnish.
Nutrition: Calories: 58 kcal, Protein: 2 g, Carbohydrates: 6 g, Fat: 4 g, Cholesterol: 0 mg, Fiber: 3 g

Whipped Ricotta Toast

Preparation Time: 15 minutes **Cooking Time:** 20 minutes **Servings:** 1
Ingredients:
- 1 1/2 c. milk ricotta cheese
- 1/4 c. extra-virgin olive oil
- 2 slices of thick-cut toast, such as sourdough
- 1/2 tsp. kosher salt

Directions:
Combine ricotta and 1/2 teaspoons of kosher salt in a food processor or blender. Blend quickly to incorporate, then carefully sprinkle in the olive oil while the machine runs. Continue processing on high speed for 2 minutes or until the ricotta is smooth and creamy. Season with pepper and spread or pipe whipped ricotta onto toast.

Nutrition: Calories: 88 kcal, Protein: 3 g, Carbohydrates: 7 g, Fat: 4 g, Cholesterol: 0 mg, Fiber: 4 g

Sikil Peak (Pumpkin Seed Salsa)

Preparation Time: 15 minutes **Cooking Time:** 20 minutes **Servings:** 1
Ingredients:
- 2 shallots, peeled

- 3/4 c. plus one tablespoon hulled raw pepitas
- 1 jalapeño, stem removed
- 4 tomatillos' husks were removed and rinsed
- 1/4 c. fresh lime juice
- 2 tsp. lime zest
- 2 cloves garlic, peeled
- 2 c. cilantro, leaves, and tender stems chopped
- 1 tsp. kosher salt, plus more to taste
- Sliced cucumbers
- Radishes
- Raw jicama sticks
- Corn tortillas
- Plantain chips

Directions:
Toast pepitas in a medium pan over medium-high heat for 5 minutes, often turning, until lightly browned; leave aside 1 tbsp for garnish. Transfer the remaining pepitas to a food processor and pulse for 30 seconds or until finely ground. It should resemble wet sand. Add tomatillos, shallots, garlic, and jalapeno to the same skillet over medium-high heat. Cook, rotating with tongs as required, until browned on both sides, approximately 5 minutes. Allow cooling slightly. Add lime zest, cilantro, juice, and salt to the food processor—pulse about 20 times or until the cilantro is wholly integrated. Process the veggies until chopped, scraping down the edges as required. Season to taste with salt and extra lime juice if desired. It should have a nutty, limey, and herbaceous flavor. Transfer to a serving dish and top with the reserved pepitas and cilantro leaves. Serve with crudités, tortilla chips, and salsa.
Nutrition: Calories: 112 kcal, Protein: 4 g, Carbohydrates: 8 g, Fat: 4 g, Cholesterol: 0 mg, Fiber: 4 g

Sweet Potato Hummus

Preparation time: 10 minutes **Cooking time:** 60 minutes **Serves** 8 to 10
Ingredients:
- 1 (15-ounce) can of chickpeas, drained
- 1-pound sweet potatoes (about 2)
- 1 teaspoon Aleppo pepper or red pepper flakes
- 4 garlic cloves, minced
- 2 tablespoons olive oil
- 2 tablespoons fresh lemon juice
- 2 teaspoons ground cumin
- Pita chips, pita bread, or fresh vegetables, for serving

Direction:
Preheat the oven to 400°F. Prick the sweet potatoes in a few places with a small, sharp knife and place them on a baking sheet. Roast until cooked through, about 1 hour, then set aside to cool. Peel the sweet potatoes and put the flesh in a blender or food processor. Add the chickpeas, garlic, olive oil, lemon juice, cumin, and ⅓ cup of water. Blend until smooth. Add the Aleppo pepper. Serve with pita chips, pita bread, or as a dip for fresh vegetables.
Nutrition: Calories: 100 | Fat: 4g | Protein: 3g | Carbohydrates: 15g| Fiber: 3g | Sugar: 2g| Sodium: 56mg

Spiced Chickpeas with Peppered Parsley

Preparation time: 10 minutes **Cooking time:** 12 minutes **Serves** 4
Ingredients:
- 1 teaspoon za'atar
- 1 (15-ounce) can of chickpeas, drained and rinsed
- 1 teaspoon Aleppo pepper
- 1 tablespoon olive oil
- ½ teaspoon ground sumac
- 1 teaspoon brown sugar
- 2 tablespoons chopped fresh parsley
- ½ teaspoon kosher salt

Direction:
Preheat the oven to 350°F. Spread the chickpeas in an even layer on an ungreased rimmed baking sheet and bake for 10 minutes or until they are dried. Remove from the oven; keep the range on. Meanwhile, whisk together the olive oil, za'atar, sumac, Aleppo pepper, brown sugar, and salt in a medium bowl until well combined. Add the warm chickpeas to the oil-spice mixture and stir until they are completely coated. Return the chickpeas to the baking sheet and spread them into an even layer. Bake for 10 to 12 minutes more, until fragrant. Transfer the chickpeas to a serving bowl, toss with the parsley, and serve.
Nutrition: Calories: 125 | Fat:5g | Protein: 5g | Carbohydrates: 16g| Fiber: 4g | Sugar: 4g| Sodium: 427mg

Roasted Plums with Honey-Yogurt Sauce

Preparation time: 5 minutes **Cooking time:** 15 minutes **Serves** 4
Ingredients:
- 6 plums, halved and pitted cooking spray
- 2 teaspoons honey
- 2 teaspoons granulated sugar
- ½ cup low-fat Greek yogurt
- 2 tablespoons chopped toasted hazelnuts

Direction:
Preheat the oven to 375°F. Line a baking sheet with parchment paper. Arrange the plums cut-side up on the baking sheet, spray with cooking spray, and sprinkle with sugar. Bake the plums in the oven until they soften and brown for about 15 minutes. Divide the plums evenly among four serving bowls and top each with a dollop of yogurt, a sprinkle of nuts, and a drizzle of honey. Serve immediately.
Nutrition: Calories: 111 | Fat: 1g | Protein: 2g | Carbohydrates: 6g| Fiber: 0g | Sugar: 6g| Sodium: 16mg

Garlic Popcorn

Preparation time: 5 minutes **Cooking time:** 0 minutes **Serves** 4
Ingredients:
- 8 cups of air-popped popcorn
- ½ teaspoon chili powder
- ⅛ teaspoon salt-free garlic powder
- ⅛ teaspoon cayenne
- ⅛ teaspoon paprika

Direction:
In a small bowl, combine the chili powder, garlic powder, paprika, and cayenne. Place the popcorn in a large bowl and toss it with the spice mixture. Serve immediately or store in an airtight container for up to 2 days.
Nutrition: Calories: 115 | Fat:5g | Protein: 7g | Carbohydrates: 42g| Fiber: 8g | Sugar: 1g| Sodium: 88mg

Zucchini Pizza Bites

Preparation time: 5 minutes **Cooking Time:** 5 minutes **Servings:** 1
Ingredients
- 1/4 cup of part-skim shredded mozzarella
- 1 medium diagonally cut zucchini.
- 1 tbsp. of quick marinara sauce
- olive oil spray
- salt and pepper

Direction:
Cut zucchini into 1/4-inch-thick slices. Season both sides with pepper and salt after gently spraying with oil. Cook the zucchini for 2 minutes on each side on the broiler or the grill, and Broil for a further minute or two after topping with the cheese and sauce. (Be careful not to overcook the cheese.)
Nutrition: Calories: 124.8 kcal, protein: 8.2 g, carbohydrates: 10.4 g, Fat: 5.7 g, Cholesterol: 12 mg, Fiber: 1.8 g

Tangy green beans

Preparation time: 10 minutes **Cooking Time:** 0 minutes **Servings:** 10
Ingredients
- 1/3 cup of diced red bell peppers
- 1 1/2 teaspoons of mustard
- 1 1/2 pounds of green beans,
- 4 1/2 teaspoons of canola oil or olive oil
- 1 1/2 teaspoons of vinegar
- 1/8 teaspoon of garlic powder
- 4 1/2 teaspoons of water
- 1/4 teaspoon of pepper
- 1/4 teaspoon of salt

Direction:
Cook the beans and red peppers in the steamer basket over water until crisp and tender. In a small mixing dish, combine the remaining ingredients. Place the beans in a serving dish and set them aside. Toss in the dressing and stir to mix it well.
Nutrition: Calories: 42 kcal, protein: 1 g, carbohydrates: 5 g, Fat: 2 g, Cholesterol: 0 mg, Fiber: 3.8 g

Corn pudding

Preparation time: 10 minutes **Cooking Time:** 20 minutes **Servings:** 8
Ingredients:
- 1/4 cup of maple syrup
- cups of coarse cornmeal (or polenta)
- 1/8 teaspoon of nutmeg
- cups of skim milk
- 1/4 teaspoon of cinnamon
- 1/8 teaspoon of clove
- 1/8 teaspoon of ginger
- 1/2 cup of raisins
- cups of water

Direction:
Bring milk and water to a boil in a saucepan. Stir in the cornmeal and keep whisking to eliminate any

lumps. Bring it back to a spot. Then reduce heat and cover for 10 to 15 minutes, stirring occasionally. Turn off the heat and add the rest of the ingredients. Allow 10 to 15 minutes for resting. Serve after a quick stir.
Nutrition: Calories: 213 kcal, protein: 6 g, carbohydrates: 45 g, Fat: 1 g, Cholesterol: 2 mg, Fiber: 1.5 g

Chili-Lime Grilled Pineapple

Preparation time: 10 minutes **Cooking Time:** 5 minutes **Servings:** 6
Ingredients
- 1 fresh pineapple
- 1 tablespoon of brown sugar
- 1 tablespoon of agave nectar or honey
- 1 tablespoon of olive oil
- 1 tablespoon of lime juice
- Dash salt
- 1-1/2 teaspoons of chili powder

Direction:
Remove the eyes from the pineapple before peeling it. Next, remove the core and cut it lengthwise into six wedges. Mix the remaining ingredients in a small bowl until well combined. Half of the glaze is brushed on the pineapple; the rest should be saved for basting. Grill covered pineapple for 2-4 minutes on each side over medium heat or broil it 4 inches from the fire until nicely browned, basting periodically with leftover glaze.
Nutrition: Calories: 97 kcal, protein: 1 g, carbohydrates: 20 g, Fat: 2 g, Cholesterol: 0 mg, Fiber: 3 g

Baked Bell Peppers

Preparation time: 10 minutes **Cooking time:** 25 minutes **Serves:** 4
Ingredients:
- 1 large red bell pepper,
- 1 large green bell pepper,
- 1 large yellow bell pepper,
- 1 large orange bell pepper,
- 1 medium red onion, sliced (optional)
- ¼ tsp acceptable sea salt
- 2 tbsp. olive oil
- Ground black pepper

Directions:
Preheat the oven to 400°F gas mark 6. Add the bell peppers and red onion (if using) to a large-sized mixing bowl. Add the olive oil and toss gently to coat. Spread out the coated bell peppers on one or two baking sheets. Make sure they aren't close to each other, or they'll steam instead of roast. Roast the bell peppers for 15 minutes, then turn them over and roast for 5 minutes more, or until slightly charred. Season with salt and pepper to taste.
Nutrition: Calories: 110; Total Fat: 7g; Saturated Fat: 1g; Cholesterol: 0mg; Sodium: 151mg; Total Carbs: 10g; Protein: 1g

Citrus Asparagus

Preparation time: 5 minutes **Cooking time:** 5 minutes **Serves:** 2
Ingredients:
- ½ lb. asparagus, woody ends trimmed
- ½ cup walnuts, finely chopped
- ½ tsp olive oil
- ½ lime, juiced and zested
- Himalayan pink salt
- Ground black pepper

Directions:
Warm the olive oil in a small-sized, nonstick frying pan over medium heat. Add the walnuts and fry for 4 minutes until fragrant and golden brown. Remove the pan from the heat and mix in the lime zest and juice. Season the walnut mixture with salt and pepper to taste, and set aside. Fill a medium-sized stockpot with water and bring it to a boil over high heat. Blanch the asparagus for 2 minutes until al dente. Discard the water and arrange the asparagus on a serving plate. Sprinkle the walnut topping over the vegetables and serve.
Nutrition: Calories: 192; Total Fat: 15g; Saturated Fat: 1g; Cholesterol: 0mg; Sodium: 10mg; Total Carbs: 11g; Net Carbs: 4g; Protein: 8g

Lemon Brussels Sprouts

Preparation time: 5 minutes **Cooking time:** 10 minutes **Serves:** 2
Ingredients:
- 1 lb. brussels sprouts, quartered
- 1 lemon juiced and zested
- 2 tsp avocado oil
- ¼ tsp garlic, crushed
- Himalayan pink salt
- Ground black pepper

Directions:
Heat the avocado oil in a medium-sized, heavy-bottom pan over medium-high heat. Add the brussels sprouts and garlic, and fry for 5 to 6 minutes until tender. Mix in the lemon juice and lemon zest, and fry for 1 minute. Season with salt and pepper to taste and serve.
Nutrition: Calories: 145; Total Fat: 6.5g; Saturated Fat: 1g; Cholesterol: 0mg; Sodium: 81mg;

Chapter 13: Smoothie and juice

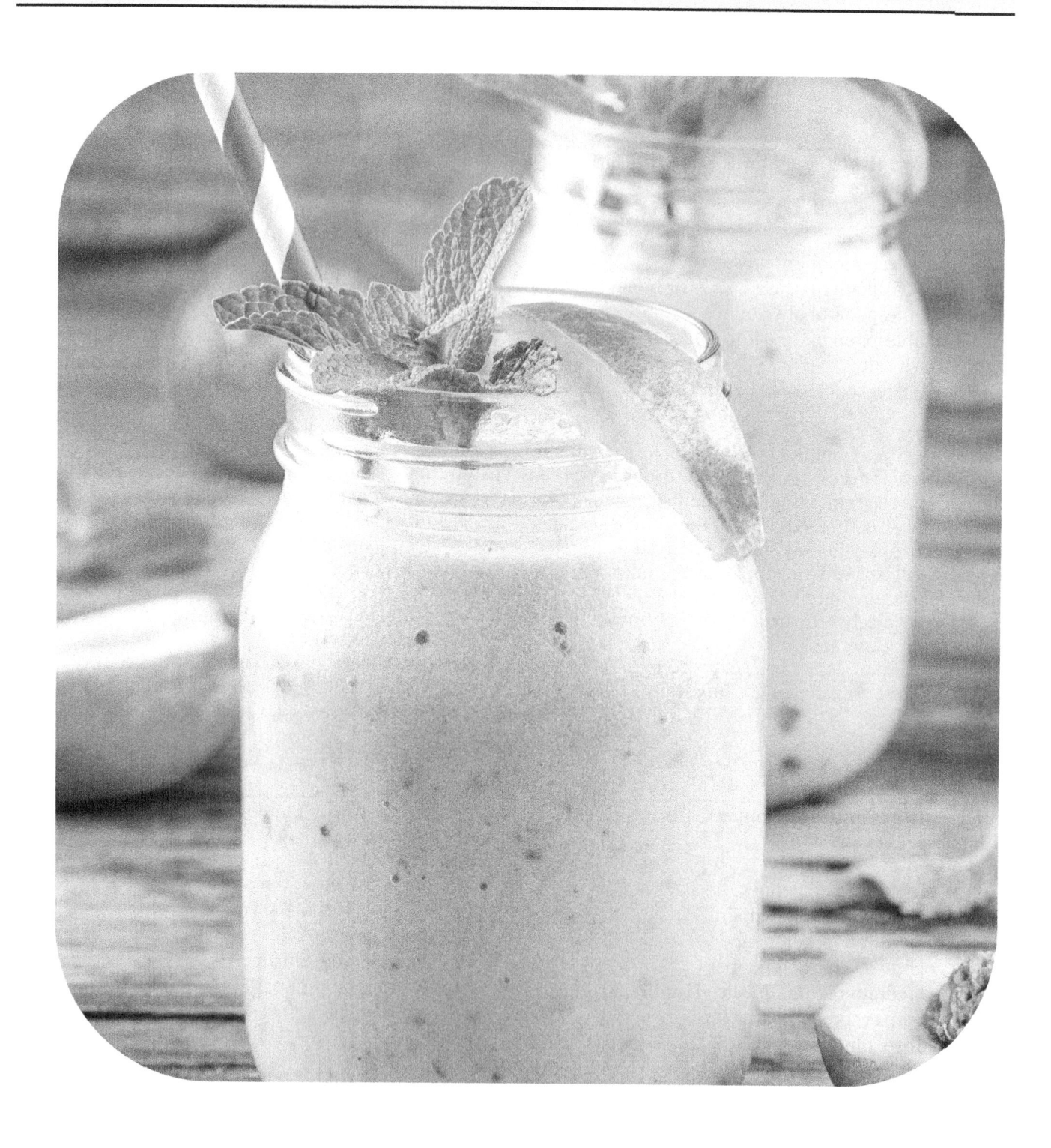

Jalapeño with Cilantro Juice

Preparation time: 5 minutes **Cooking time:** 0 minutes **Serves** 1
Ingredients:
- 1 orange
- ¼ fresh pineapple
- ½ handful cilantro
- ½ small jalapeno, seeded

Direction:
Peel the pineapple and orange and juice them with the jalapeno and cilantro in a juicer. Pour the juice into a glass and serve immediately.
Nutrition: Calories: 71| Fat: 0g | Protein: 1g | Carbohydrates: 20g | Sugar: 15mg

Grapy Weight Loss Juice

Preparation time: 5 minutes **Cooking time:** 0 minutes **Serves** 1
Ingredients:
- 1 ruby grapefruit
- 1 orange
- 2 carrots, ½-inch (1 cm) piece of ginger

Direction:
All ingredients must be washed and peeled. Juice immediately after passing through a juicer.
Nutrition: Calories: 25| Fat: 0g | Protein: 0g | Carbohydrates: 6g | Sugar: 3mg

Icy Orange Juice with Lemon

Preparation time: 5 minutes **Cooking time:** 0 minutes **Serves** 1
Ingredients:
- ½ young cabbage
- 1 small carrot
- 3 oranges, peeled
- ½ lemon juice, a thumb size piece of ginger
- Ice cubes

Direction:
Juice the carrots, ginger, cabbage, and oranges using a juicer. Pour into a glass, top with lemon juice, and serve.
Nutrition: Calories: 25| Fat: 0g | Protein: 0g | Carbohydrates: 6g | Sugar: 3mg

Fruity Mixed Juice

Preparation time: 5 minutes **Cooking time:** 0 minutes **Serves** 1
Ingredients:
- 4 rounds of pineapple
- 1 grapefruit (juice of 1 grapefruit)
- 1 cup of water

Direction:
Peel and cut the pineapple into rounds. Pass through a juicer with the grapefruit. Pour the juice into a tall glass, add 1 cup of water, and stir well before drinking.
Nutrition: Calories: 84| Fat: 0g | Protein: 2g | Carbohydrates: 21g | Sugar: 18mg

Avocado Mix with Ice

Preparation time: 5 minutes **Cooking time:** 0 minutes **Serves** 1
Ingredients:
- ½ ripe avocado
- ½ small pineapple
- 2 apples, cored, quartered
- ½ stick celery
- 1 small handful of spinach leaves
- 1 small piece of peeled lime
- ½ of a medium cucumber
- Ice cubes

Direction:
Cut the apples into quarters after coring them. Juice the cucumber, lime, spinach, pineapple, and celery in a juicer. Put the avocado in a blender after peeling it. Add a few ice cubes and process for 20 to 30 seconds, or until smooth. Combine the avocado mixture and the extracted juice in a glass, stir well, and drink immediately.
Nutrition: Calories: 187| Fat: 8g | Protein: 2g | Carbohydrates: 32g | Sugar: 20mg

Apple-Carrot Juice

Preparation time: 5 minutes **Cooking time:** 0 minutes **Serves:** 2
Ingredients:
- 6 carrots
- 4 apple 2-inch (5 cm) piece of fresh root ginger

Direction:
As needed, peel, cut, deseed, and chop the ingredients. Put a container beneath the juicer's

spout. Feed the ingredients through the juicer one at a time, in the order listed. Pour the juice into glasses and serve.
Nutrition: Calories: 262| Fat: 0g | Protein: 1g | Carbohydrates: 33g | Sugar: 20mg

Cinnamon with Potatoes Juice

Preparation time: 5 minutes **Cooking time:** 0 minutes **Serves** 1
Ingredients:
- 6 large carrots
- 1½ sweet potatoes
- 2 red apple dash of ground cinnamon

Direction:
As needed, peel, cut, deseed, and chop the ingredients. Put a container beneath the juicer's spout. Feed the ingredients through the juicer one at a time, in the order listed. Pour the juice into glasses and serve.
Nutrition: Calories: 355| Fat: 0g | Protein: 81g | Carbohydrates: 1g | Sugar: 236mg

Mint lime with cucumber and carrot

Preparation time: 10 minutes **Cooking time:** 0 minutes **Serves:** 2
Ingredients:
- 8 carrots
- 2 cucumbers
- 4 apples
- 1 lime
- Large handful of fresh mint
- 2-inch (5 cm) piece of fresh root ginger

Direction:
As needed, peel, cut, deseed, and chop the ingredients. Put a container beneath the juicer's spout. Feed the ingredients through the juicer one at a time, in the order listed. Pour the juice into glasses and serve.
Nutrition: Calories: 267| Fat: 0g | Protein: 60g | Carbohydrates: 1g | Sugar: 120mg

Kale-Banana smoothie

Preparation Time: 5 minutes **Cooking time:** 0 minutes **Serves:** 2
Ingredients:
- 1 banana, halved and frozen
- 1 cup chopped cucumber
- 2 cups chopped kale
- 2 tablespoons ground flaxseed
- 1 cup coconut milk
- ½ cup water

Direction:
Combine the banana, cucumber, kale, flaxseed, coconut milk, and water in a blender. Blend until smooth on high speed. Divide evenly between two cups and serve.
Nutrition: Calories: 488; Total Fat: 38.7g; Sugars: 15.3g; Carbohydrates: 38.7g; Fiber: 4.7g; Protein: 6.1g; Sodium: 45.7mg

Apple Tart smoothie

Preparation Time: 5 minutes **Cooking time:** 0 minutes **Serves:** 2
Ingredients:
- 1 red apple, chopped and frozen
- 2 cups chopped Boston lettuce
- 1 avocado, chopped and frozen
- ½ cup walnuts
- 1 tablespoon apple cider vinegar
- 1½ cups water

Direction:
Combine the apple, lettuce, avocado, walnuts, vinegar, and water in a blender. Blend until smooth on high speed. Divide evenly between two cups and serve.
Nutrition: Calories: 407; Total Fat: 34.1g; Sugars: 11.4g; Carbohydrates: 26.4g; Fiber: 11.5g; Protein: 7.4g; Sodium: 11.3mg

Kiwi, Zucchini, and Pear smoothie

Preparation Time: 5 minutes **Cooking time:** 0 minutes **Serves** 2
Ingredients:
- 2 kiwis, peeled, chopped, and frozen
- 1 cup chopped zucchini
- 1 pear, chopped and frozen
- 1 cup fresh spinach
- 1½ cups unsweetened almond milk

Direction:
Put the kiwi, zucchini, pear, spinach, and almond milk in a blender. Blend on high speed until smooth. Divide evenly between 2 cups and enjoy!
Nutrition: Calories: 121; Total Fat: 3g; Sugars:

13.6g; Carbohydrates: 23.4g; Fiber: 6.4g; Protein: 3.3g; Sodium: 165mg

Green Mango smoothie

Preparation time: 5 minutes **Cooking time:** 0 minutes **Serves:** 2
Ingredients:
- 1 cup frozen mango chunks
- 2 cups chopped radish greens
- 1 avocado, peeled and pitted
- 2 tablespoons chia seeds
- 1 cup full-fat plain Greek yogurt
- 1½ cups water

Direction:
Put the mango, radish greens, avocado, chia seeds, yogurt, and water in a blender. Blend on high speed until smooth. Divide evenly between 2 cups and enjoy!
Nutrition: Calories: 440; Total Fat: 26.8g; Sugars: 12.9g; Carbohydrates: 37g; Fiber: 16.2g; Protein: 17.4g; Sodium: 88.3mg

Carroty Breakfast Grind

Preparation time: 10 minutes **Cooking time:** 0 minutes **Serving:** 3
Ingredients:
- 2 lemons, peeled, seeded, and quartered
- 2 carrots, chopped
- 2 apples, peeled and quartered
- 2 beets, trimmed and chopped
- 2 cups fresh spinach

Direction:
Press all ingredients through a juicer into a glass or pitcher.
Nutrition: Calories: 115 Fat: 0.5 g Protein: 2 g Carbohydrates: 29 g Sugar: 19 mg

Juicy Morning Blaster

Preparation time: 10 minutes **Cooking time:** 0 minutes **Serving:** 2
Ingredients:
- 1 whole cucumber
- 2 green apples
- 3 celery stalks
- 2 oranges
- 1/2 bunch of spinach

Direction:
Wash all produce. Quarter apples and remove all seeds. Peel oranges and remove all seeds. Roll spinach leaves to fit into your juicer. Blend all produce together in your juicer. This can be blended with or served over ice if desired. Stir and drink immediately.
Nutrition: Calories: 231 Fat: 1 g Protein: 6 g Carbohydrates: 56 g Sugar: 21 mg

Fresh Morning Juice

Preparation time: 10 minutes **Cooking time:** 0 minutes **Serving:** 2
Ingredients:
- 1 cup pineapple, cut into chunks
- 1 green apple, quartered
- 1 cup fresh spinach
- 1 leaf kale
- 1 avocado, peeled and pitted

Direction:
Press all ingredients through a juicer into a large glass. Stir before serving.
Nutrition: Calories: 286 Fat: 15 g Protein: 3 g Carbohydrates: 41 g Sugar: 28 mg

Early-Berry Juice

Preparation time: 10 minutes **Cooking time:** 0 minutes **Serving:** 4
Ingredients:
- 3 blood oranges
- 3 large apples
- 3 large pears
- 2 cups fresh cranberries

Direction:
Prepare your pears and apples by cutting them into small chunks that your juicer can easily handle. Peel and cut your oranges into sixths. Add the apples, oranges, and pears to the juicer, then stir in the cranberries. Store in an airtight container for up to a week before serving.
Nutrition: Calories: 329 Fat: 1 g Protein: 3 g Carbohydrates: 85 g Sugar: 49 mg

Rise and Shine Morning Juice

Preparation time: 10 minutes **Cooking time:** 0 minutes **Serving:** 2
Ingredients:
- 1 beet, peeled
- 2 carrots, roughly peeled
- 1 cup pineapple
- 1 lemon

Directions:

Cut veggies and fruit into pieces small enough to fit in the juicer. Remove visible seeds from the lemon but keep peeling on it for extra zip. Slowly add ingredients to the juicer until you've juiced it all! Enjoy chilled.
Nutrition: Calories: 114 Fat: 0.3 g Protein: 2 g Carbohydrates: 29 g Sugar: 23 mg

Green Monster

Preparation Time: 5 minutes **Cooking time:** 0 minutes **Serves:** 2
Ingredients:
- 1 avocado, peeled and pitted
- 2 cups chopped kale
- 3 tablespoons hulled hemp seeds
- 1 cup frozen grapes
- 1 cup coconut milk
- ½ cup water

Direction:
Put the kale, avocado, grapes, hemp seeds, coconut milk, and water in a blender. Blend on high speed until smooth. Divide evenly between 2 cups and enjoy!
Nutrition: Calories: 554; Total Fat: 46.4g; Sugars: 12.3g; Carbohydrates: 33.1g; Fiber: 8.8g; Protein: 12g; Sodium: 52.1mg

Orange Sunrise

Preparation Time: 5 minutes **Cooking time:** 0 minutes **Serves:** 2
Ingredients:
- 1 cup frozen mango chunks
- ½ cup rolled oats
- 1 cup full-fat plain Greek yogurt
- 2 tablespoons cashew butter
- 2 cups unsweetened almond milk

Direction:
Put the mango, oats, yogurt, cashew butter, and almond milk in a blender. Blend on high speed until smooth. Divide evenly between 2 cups and enjoy!
Nutrition: Calories: 441; Total Fat: 19.8g; Sugars: 12.2g; Carbohydrates: 45.3g; Fiber: 6.9g; Protein: 20.8g; Sodium: 212mg

Purple Passion

Preparation Time: 5 minutes **Cooking time:** 0 minutes **Serves:** 2
Ingredients:
- 1 avocado, peeled and pitted
- 2 plums, diced and frozen
- 1½ cups full-fat cottage cheese
- 1 cup frozen blackberries
- 1½ cups unsweetened almond milk

Direction:
Put the plums, blackberries, avocado, cottage cheese, and almond milk in a blender. Blend on high speed until smooth. Divide evenly between 2 cups and enjoy!
Nutrition: Calories: 414; Total Fat: 24.8g; Sugars: 15.2g; Carbohydrates: 29.9g; Fiber: 12.2g; Protein: 23g; Sodium: 742mg

Chapter 14: Dessert

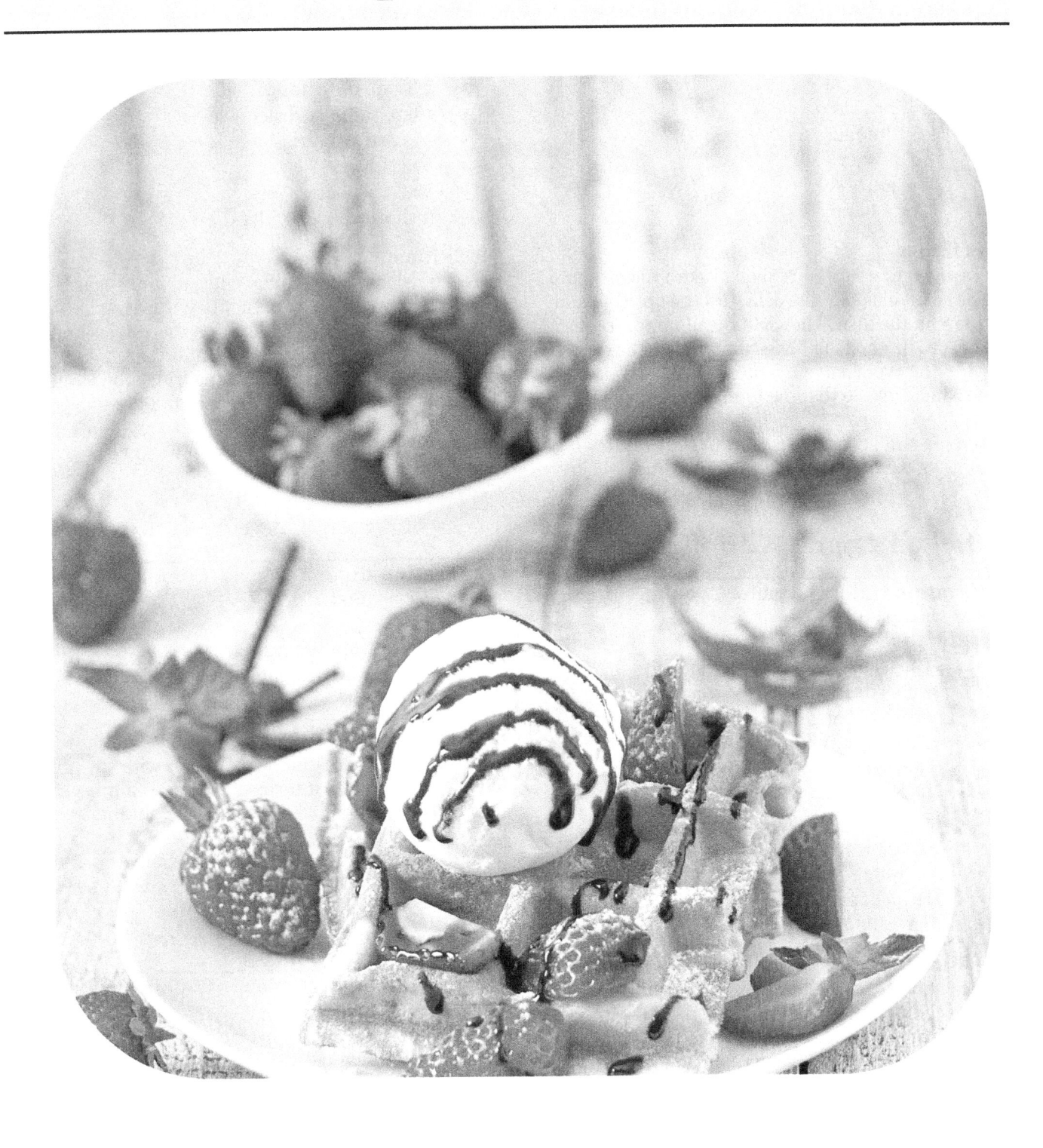

Apricot Crisp

Preparation time: 5 mins **Cooking time:** 25 mins **Servings:** 2
Ingredients:
- 1 tsp. olive oil
- 1 lb. apricots
- ½ c. almonds
- 1 Tbsp. oats
- 1 tsp. anise seeds
- 2 Tbsp. honey

Directions:
Set the oven to 350° Fahrenheit. Take a pie dish and brush the oil inside of the dish. Cut the apricots and put them in the dish. Then add the almonds, seeds, and oats to it. Pour the honey on top. Put the dish in the oven for twenty-five minutes. Take it out of the range when you see that the topping has turned golden. Serve warm.
Nutrition: Calories 134; Fat 6g; Carbohydrates 17g; Proteins 3g; Cholesterol 0mg; Sodium 1mg

Baked Apples with Almonds

Preparation time: 15 minutes **Cooking time:** 1-hour **Servings:** 4
Ingredients:
- 3 Tbsp. almonds, chopped roughly
- 1 c. cherries
- 2 Tbsp. wheat germ
- 2 Tbsp. brown sugar
- ½ tsp. cinnamon powder
- 1/8 tsp. nutmeg powder
- 4 apples
- ½ c. apple juice
- ¼ c. water
- 2 Tbsp. dark honey
- 2 tsp. walnut oil

Directions:
Set the oven to 350° Fahrenheit. Put the nutmeg, sugar, cinnamon, wheat germ, cherries, and almonds in a bowl. Give it a mix, and keep it aside for now. Core the apples from the center and add the cherry mix to them. Take a baking dish and place the apples on the dish in an upright position. Add apple juice with some water to the dish. Drizzle oil and honey over the apples and cover the dish with aluminum foil. Put the dish in the oven for an hour. Then take them out and serve warm.
Nutrition: Calories 200; Fat 4g; Carbohydrates 39g; Proteins 2g; Cholesterol 0mg; Sodium 7mg

Berries with Balsamic Vinegar

Preparation time: 5 minutes **Cooking time:** 15 minutes **Servings:** 2
Ingredients:
- ¼ c. balsamic vinegar
- 2 Tbsp. brown sugar
- 1 tsp. vanilla extract
- ½ c. strawberries
- ½ c. blueberries
- ½ c. raspberries
- 2 shortbread biscuits

Directions:
Take a bowl and add vanilla, vinegar, and sugar. Whisk them well. Take another bowl and put all the berries in it. Drizzle the vinegar on the berries and let them sit for fifteen minutes. Drain the excess vinegar from the berries. Keep them in the fridge for a while. Serve them with the shortbread biscuit.
Nutrition: Calories 176; Fat 4g; Carbohydrates 33g; Proteins 2g; Cholesterol 5mg; Sodium 56mg

Cookie Cream Shake

Preparation time: 10 minutes **Cooking time:** 0 minutes **Servings:** 2
Ingredients:
- 1 1/3 c. vanilla soy milk
- 3 c. vanilla ice cream
- 4 chocolate wafer cookies

Directions:
In a food processor, add the ice cream with soy milk. Blend everything till it turns into a smooth mix. Then add the cookies and blend again. Take out the smoothie in glasses and serve.
Nutrition: Calories 270; Fat 3g; Carbohydrates 52g; Proteins 9g; Cholesterol 270mg; Sodium 244mg

Creamy Fruit Dessert

Preparation time: 15 minutes **Cooking time:** 0 minutes **Servings:** 2
Ingredients:
- 6 oz. cream cheese
- ½ c. yogurt
- 1 tsp. sugar
- 1 tsp. vanilla extract
- 10 oz. mandarin oranges, cut into pieces
- 10 oz. peaches, diced
- 8 oz. pineapple, cubed
- 4 Tbsp. shredded coconut

Directions:

Take a bowl and put all the ingredients except the fruit in it. Then beat them with an electric mixer till it becomes smooth. Mix all the fruits in a bowl and pour the cream mixture over them. Gently fold it. Now place this bowl in the fridge and leave it there for a while to get chilled. Take out in a bowl and sprinkle the shredded coconut on top of it and serve.
Nutrition: Calories 206; Fat 2g; Carbohydrates 41g; Proteins 6g; Cholesterol 3mg; Sodium 241mg

Cheddar Cake

Preparation Time: 10 minutes **Cooking Time:** 45 minutes **Servings:** 8
Ingredients:
- 2 eggs
- ¼ cup coconut flour
- 14.5 oz ricotta
- ½ cup erythritol
- Pinch of salt

Directions:
Preheat the stove to 350° F. In a bowl, whisk eggs, add the other ingredients and blend until all around joined. Pour the player into the lubed baking container. Bake in a broiler for 45 minutes. Allow cooling. Slice and Servings.
Nutrition: •Calories 90 •Fat 5 g •Sugars 3 g •Sugar 0.3 g •Protein 7 g •Cholesterol 3 mg

Yogurt Cheesecake

Preparation time: 15 minutes **Cooking time:** 35 minutes **Serving:** 4
Ingredients:
- 1¼ cup fat-free Greek yogurt
- 2 tablespoons arrowroot starch
- 1½ egg whites
- ½ cup cocoa powder
- ½ teaspoon organic vanilla extract

Direction:
Preheat the baking oven to 350° F and grease a cake pan. Meanwhile, add everything to a bowl and mix well. Pour the mixture into the cake pan and bake for about 35 minutes. Take out and set aside to cool. Refrigerate for three to four hours, slice, and serve.
Nutrition: Calories: 180 Fat: 5.6g Sat Fat: 3.3g Carbohydrates: 26.8g Fiber: 3.3g Sugar: 16.4g Protein: 11.7g

Sweet potato and pumpkin pie

Preparation time: 10 minutes **Cooking time:** 60 minutes **Serving:** 8
Ingredients:
- 1 sweet potato peeled and cooked
- 1 buttercup squash, peeled, seeded, and cooked
- ½ cup silken tofu
- ½ cup soy milk
- ¼ cup egg whites
- ¼ cup rye flour
- ½ tsp. each clove, cinnamon, nutmeg, and vanilla extract
- 1 tsp. freshly grated ginger
- 1 tsp. orange zest
- 3 tbsp. honey
- 1 frozen pre-made 9-inch pie shell

Direction:
Heat the oven to 300° F. Puree the sweet potato and squash in a food processor. Place in a large bowl. Add the remaining and mix until smooth and well-combined. Place the pie shell on a sheet pan. Pour the mixture into the pie shell and bake for 45 to 55 minutes or until the internal temperature is 180° F.
Nutrition: Calories 210 Protein 5g Carbohydrate 34g Dietary fiber 4g Sugars 7g Fat 6g Sodium 109mg

Crepes with strawberries and cream cheese

Preparation time: 15 minutes **Cooking time:** 10 minutes **Serving:** 4
Ingredients:
- 4 tbsp. cream cheese softened
- 2 tbsp. sifted powdered sugar
- 2 tsp. vanilla extract
- 2 prepackaged crepes, each about
- 8 inches in diameter
- 8 strawberries, hulled and sliced
- 1 tsp. powdered sugar for garnish
- 2 tbsp. caramel sauce, warmed

Direction:
Heat the oven to 325° F. Lightly coat a baking dish with cooking spray. In a mixing bowl, blend the cream cheese until smooth using an electric mixer. Add the powdered sugar and vanilla. Mix well. Spread ½ of the cream cheese mixture on each crepe, leaving ½-inch around the edge. Top with 2 tbsp of strawberries. Roll up each crepe and place seam-side down in the prepared baking dish. Bake until lightly browned (about 10 minutes). Cut the crepes in half.

Transfer to four individual serving plates.
Nutrition: Calories 143 Protein 3g Carbohydrate 17g Dietary Fiber 0.5g Fat 7g Sugars 7g Sodium 161mg

Apple-Berry Cobbler

Preparation time: 55 minutes **Cooking time:** 40 minutes **Serving:** 6
Ingredients:
The Filling:
- 1 cup fresh raspberries
- 1 cup fresh blueberries
- 2 cups chopped apples
- 2 tbsp. Turbinado or brown sugar
- ½ tsp. ground cinnamon
- 1 tsp. lemon zest
- 2 tsp. lemon juice
- 1½ tbsp. corn starch

The Topping:
- 1 large egg
- ¼ cup soy milk
- ¼ tsp. Salt
- ½ tsp. vanilla
- 1½ tbsp. turbinado or brown sugar
- ¾ cup whole-wheat pastry flour

Direction:
Oven temperature set to 350 °F. Cooking spray should be lightly applied to six individual oven-safe ramekins. In a medium bowl, combine the apples, raspberries, blueberries, sugar, cinnamon, and lemon juice. To blend evenly, stir. Stir in the cornstarch after adding it. Place aside. In a another dish, combine the egg white and whisk until just beaten. Add the pastry flour, sugar, salt, vanilla, and soy milk. Stir well to combine. In the ramekins that have been ready, distribute the fruit mixture evenly. Give each the topping to eat. Place the ramekins on a large baking sheet and in the oven. Bake until the topping is golden and the filling is soft (about 30 minutes).
Nutrition: Calories 119 Protein 3.5g Carbohydrate24 g Dietary Fiber 4g Sugars 12 g Fat 0g Sodium 114mg

Mint chocolate dessert with banana

Preparation time: 5 minutes **Cooking time:** 0 minutes **Serving:** 4
Ingredients:
- 3 bananas, sliced and frozen
- 4 tablespoons unsweetened cocoa powder
- ½ teaspoon peppermint extract
- 2 to 3 tablespoons nonfat or low-fat milk (optional)

Direction:
Remove the frozen bananas from the freezer and let them stand for about 5 minutes. Add the banana, cocoa, and peppermint extract to a food processor and pulse until the banana slices are finely chopped. Then purée until the mixture resembles soft-serve ice cream, adding the milk (if using).
Nutrition: Calories: 92 Fat: 1g Protein: 2g Carbohydrates: 23g Fiber: 4g Sugar: 11g Sodium: 2mg

Baked Apples with Cherries and Almonds

Preparation time: 20 minutes **Cooking time:** 60 minutes **Serving:** 6
Ingredients:
- 1/3 cup dried cherries, coarsely chopped
- 6 small Golden Delicious apples
- 3 tbsp. chopped almonds
- 1 tbsp. wheat germ
- 1 tbsp. Firmly packed brown sugar
- ½ cup apple juice
- ½ tsp. ground cinnamon
- 1/8 tsp. ground nutmeg
- 2 tsp. walnut oil or canola oil
- ¼ cup water
- 2 tbsp. dark honey

Direction:
Preheat the oven to 350 °F. Cherries, almonds, wheat germ, brown sugar, cinnamon, and nutmeg should all be combined together thoroughly in a small basin. Place aside. If you'd prefer, the apples can be left unpeeled. Using a vegetable peeler or a sharp knife, remove the peel in a circular motion from each apple, skipping every other row so that rows of apple flesh alternate with rows of skin. Core each apple starting at the stem end and stopping ¾ inch from the bottom. Then, evenly distribute the cherry mixture among the apples, gently pressing it into each cavity. In a sturdy, oven-safe frying pan or small baking dish that is just big enough to hold them, arrange the apples upright. Water and apple juice should be added to the pan. Spread the apples with the honey and oil, and then tightly wrap the pan with aluminum foil. Bake the apples until they are soft when pricked with a knife (50 to 60 minutes).
Nutrition: Calories 200 Protein 2g Carbohydrate 39g Dietary Fiber 5g Sugars 8g Fat 4g Sodium 7mg

Fruit Cake

Preparation time: 20 minutes **Cooking time:** 35 minutes **Serving:** 9
Ingredients:
- 2 cups of various chopped dried fruits, such as figs, dates, cherries, or currants
- ½ cup unsweetened apple sauce
- ¼ cup sugar
- 1 egg
- ½ cup crushed pineapple packed in juice, drained
- Zest and juice of 1 medium orange
- Zest and juice of 1 lemon
- ½ cup unsweetened apple juice
- ¼ cup flaxseed flour
- 2 tbsp. real vanilla extract
- ½ cup rolled oats
- 1 cup whole-wheat pastry flour
- ½ tsp. baking powder
- ½ tsp. baking soda
- ½ cup crushed or chopped walnuts

Direction:
Preheat the oven to 325°F. Combine the dried fruit, applesauce, pineapple, fruit zests and juices, and vanilla in a medium bowl. Let the mixture soak for 15 to 20 minutes. Line the bottom of a 9 x 4-inch pan with parchment paper. Whisk together the sugar, oats, flour, baking soda, and baking powder in a large bowl. Add the fruit and liquid mixture to the dry ingredients and stir to combine. Add the egg and walnuts and stir to combine. Bake for an hour, or until a toothpick inserted in the center comes out clean, after pouring the mixture into the loaf pan. Before taking the fruitcake from the pan, allow it to cool for 30 minutes.
Nutrition: Calories 229 Protein 5g Carbohydrate 41g Dietary fiber 5g Sugar 5g Fat 3g Sodium 117mg

Carrot cookies

Preparation time: 5 minutes **Cooking time:** 20 minutes Serving: 6
Ingredients:
- 2 eggs
- ½ cup apple sauce
- ½ cup brown sugar
- ½ cup sugar
- ½ cup oil
- 1 teaspoon vanilla extract
- 2 cups old-fashioned rolled oats
- 1 cup flour
- 1 cup whole-wheat flour
- 1 teaspoon baking powder
- 1 teaspoon baking soda
- ¼ teaspoon salt
- 1 teaspoon ground cinnamon
- ½ teaspoon ground nutmeg
- ½ teaspoon ground ginger
- 1½ cups finely grated carrots
- 1 cup raisins or golden raisins

Direction:
Preheat the oven to 350°F. Mix the applesauce with the eggs, oil, sugars, and vanilla in a bowl. Stir in all the dry ingredients. Mix well, then fold in the carrots and raisins. Drop a tablespoon of cookie dough on a cookie sheet. Add more cookies drop by drop. Bake the cookies 15 minutes until golden brown. Serve.
Nutrition: Calories 124 Fat 5g Sodium 32mg Carbs 31g Fiber 0.3g Sugar 1g Protein 5.7g

Hot chocolate pudding

Preparation time: 15 minutes **Cooking time:** 10 minutes **Serving**: 6
Ingredients:
- 2 tbsp. corn starch
- 3 tbsp. brewed espresso
- 1 tbsp. ground flaxseeds (flax meal)
- 2/3 cup sugar, divided
- 2 ¼ cups skim milk, divided
- 1/8 tsp. salt
- 2/3 cup unsweetened cocoa powder
- 1 tsp. vanilla extract

Direction:
With a fork, stir the warm espresso into the ground flaxseeds (flax meal) in a medium bowl. Place aside. In a medium saucepan, combine 1 1/2 cups milk, 1/3 cup sugar, and salt. Over medium heat, bring to a simmer while stirring occasionally. In the meantime, combine the remaining cornstarch, cocoa powder, and 1/3 cup sugar in a medium bowl. After that, mix the remaining 3/4 cup milk until well combined. Mix the cocoa mixture with the milk mixture that is boiling. Return the mixture to the pan and cook it over medium heat, whisking continually, until it thickens and becomes glossy (about 3 minutes). Get rid of the heat. One cup of the hot cocoa mixture should be incorporated with the beaten flaxseeds. Stirring continually, add this mixture to the pan and heat over low heat until it steams and thickens (about 2 minutes). Keep the mixture from boiling.
Nutrition: Calories 169 Protein 5g Carbohydrate 35g Dietary fiber 2g Sugar 22g Fat 1g Sodium 86mg

Roasted plums with walnut crumble

Preparation Time: 5 Minutes **Cooking Time:** 25 Minutes **Serves** 4
Ingredients:
- ¼ cup honey
- ¼ cup freshly squeezed orange juice
- 4 large plums, halved and pitted
- ¼ cup whole-wheat pastry flour
- 1 tablespoon pure maple sugar
- 1 tablespoon nuts, coarsely chopped
- 1½ teaspoons olive oil
- ½ cup plain Greek yogurt

Direction:
Preheat the oven to 400°F. Combine the honey and orange juice in a square baking dish. Place the plums, cut-side down, in the dish. Roast for about 15 minutes, then turn the plums over and roast for 10 minutes, or until tender and juicy. Mix well in a medium bowl. Combine the flour, maple sugar, nuts, and olive oil. Spread on a small baking sheet and bake alongside the plums, tossing once, until golden brown, about 5 minutes. Set aside until the plums have finished cooking. Serve the plums drizzled with pan juices and topped with the nut crumble and a dollop of yogurt.
Nutrition: Calories: 175| Total fat: 3g| Saturated fat: 0g| Cholesterol: 0mg| Sodium: 10mg| Potassium: 215mg| Total Carbohydrates: 36g| Fiber: 2g| Sugars: 28g| Protein: 4g|

Mascarpone and honey figs

Preparation Time: 5 Minutes **Cooking Time:** 5 Minutes **Serves** 4
Ingredients:
- ¼ cup mascarpone cheese
- 8 fresh figs, halved
- ⅓ cup walnuts, chopped
- 1 tablespoon honey
- ¼ teaspoon flaked sea salt

Direction:
For three to five minutes, toast the walnuts in a pan over medium heat while turning frequently. Place the figs on a tray or platter with the cut side up. Each fig's sliced side should have a little depression made with your finger and filled with mascarpone cheese. Add a little amount of walnuts, a drizzle of honey, and a dash of sea salt.
Nutrition: Calories: 201 Total fat: 13g| Saturated fat: 4g| Cholesterol: 18mg| Sodium: 105mg| Potassium: 230mg| Total Carbohydrates: 24g| Fiber: 3g| Sugars: 18g| Protein: 3g

Chocolate "Mousse" with Greek Yogurt and Berries

Preparation Time: 30 minutes **Cooking Time:** 5 Minutes **Serves** 4
Ingredients:
- 2 cups plain Greek yogurt
- ¼ cup heavy cream
- ¼ cup pure maple syrup
- 3 tablespoons unsweetened cocoa powder
- 2 teaspoons vanilla extract
- ¼ teaspoon kosher salt
- 1 cup fresh mixed berries
- ¼ cup chocolate chips

Direction:
Place the yogurt, cream, maple syrup, cocoa powder, vanilla, and salt in the bowl of a stand mixer, or use a large bowl with an electric hand mixer. Mix at medium-high speed until fluffy, about 5 minutes. Spoon evenly among 4 bowls and put in the refrigerator to set for at least 15 minutes. Serve each bowl with ¼ cup mixed berries and 1 tablespoon chocolate chips.
Nutrition: Calories: 300| Total fat: 11g| Saturated fat: 6g| Cholesterol: 27mg| Sodium: 60mg| Potassium: 295mg| Total Carbohydrates: 35g| Fiber: 3g| Sugars: 29g| Protein: 16g

Meringues with Strawberries, Mint, and Toasted Coconut

Preparation Time: 25 Minutes **Cooking Time:** 1 Hour, 30 Minutes **Serves** 6
Ingredients:
- 4 large egg whites
- 8 ounces strawberries, diced
- ¼ cup fresh mint, chopped
- 1 teaspoon vanilla extract
- ½ teaspoon cream of tartar
- ¾ cup sugar
- ¼ cup unsweetened shredded coconut, toasted

Direction:
Preheat the oven to 225°F. Line 2 baking sheets with parchment paper. Place the egg whites, vanilla, and cream of tartar in the bowl of a stand mixer (or use a large bowl with an electric hand mixer)| beat at

medium speed until soft peaks form, about 2 to 3 minutes. Increase to high speed and gradually add the sugar, beating until stiff peaks form and the mixture looks shiny and smooth for about 2 to 3 minutes. Using a spatula or spoon, drop ⅓ cup of meringue onto a Prepared baking sheet| smooth out and make shapelier as desired. Make 12 dollops, 6 per sheet, leaving at least 1 inch between dollops. 4 Bake for 1½ hours, rotating baking sheets between top and bottom, front and back, halfway through. After 1½ hours, turn off the oven, but keep the door closed. Leave the meringues in the oven for an additional 30 minutes. You can leave the meringues in the oven even longer (or overnight), or you may let them finish cooling to room temperature. 5 Combine the strawberries, mint, and coconut in a medium bowl. Serve 2 meringues per person topped with the fruit mixture.

Nutrition: Calories: 150| Total fat: 2g| Saturated fat: 2g| Cholesterol: 0mg| Sodium: 40mg| Potassium: 165mg| Total Carbohydrates: 29g| Fiber: 1g| Sugars: 27g| Protein: 3g

Pistachio-Stuffed Dates

Preparation Time: 10 Minutes **Cooking Time:** 5 Minutes **Serves** 4
Ingredients:
- ½ cup unsalted pistachios shelled
- ¼ teaspoon kosher salt
- 8 Medjool dates, pitted

Direction:
In a food processor, add the pistachios and salt. Process until combined with chunky nut butter, 3 to 5 minutes. Split open the dates and spoon the pistachio nut butter into each half.

Nutrition: Calories: 220| Total fat: 7g| Saturated fat: 1g| Cholesterol: 0mg| Sodium: 70mg| Potassium: 490mg| Total Carbohydrates: 41g| Fiber: 5g| Sugars: 33g| Protein: 4g

Conversion Tables of the Various Units of Measurement

COOKING CONVERSION CHART

Measurement

CUP	ONCES	MILLILITERS	TABLESPOONS
8 cup	64 oz	1895 ml	128
6 cup	48 oz	1420 ml	96
5 cup	40 oz	1180 ml	80
4 cup	32 oz	960 ml	64
2 cup	16 oz	480 ml	32
1 cup	8 oz	240 ml	16
3/4 cup	6 oz	177 ml	12
2/3 cup	5 oz	158 ml	11
1/2 cup	4 oz	118 ml	8
3/8 cup	3 oz	90 ml	6
1/3 cup	2.5 oz	79 ml	5.5
1/4 cup	2 oz	59 ml	4
1/8 cup	1 oz	30 ml	3
1/16 cup	1/2 oz	15 ml	1

Temperature

FAHRENHEIT	CELSIUS
100 °F	37 °C
150 °F	65 °C
200 °F	93 °C
250 °F	121 °C
300 °F	150 °C
325 °F	160 °C
350 °F	180 °C
375 °F	190 °C
400 °F	200 °C
425 °F	220 °C
450 °F	230 °C
500 °F	260 °C
525 °F	274 °C
550 °F	288 °C

Weight

IMPERIAL	METRIC
1/2 oz	15 g
1 oz	29 g
2 oz	57 g
3 oz	85 g
4 oz	113 g
5 oz	141 g
6 oz	170 g
8 oz	227 g
10 oz	283 g
12 oz	340 g
13 oz	369 g
14 oz	397 g
15 oz	425 g
1 lb	453 g

30 Day Meal Plan

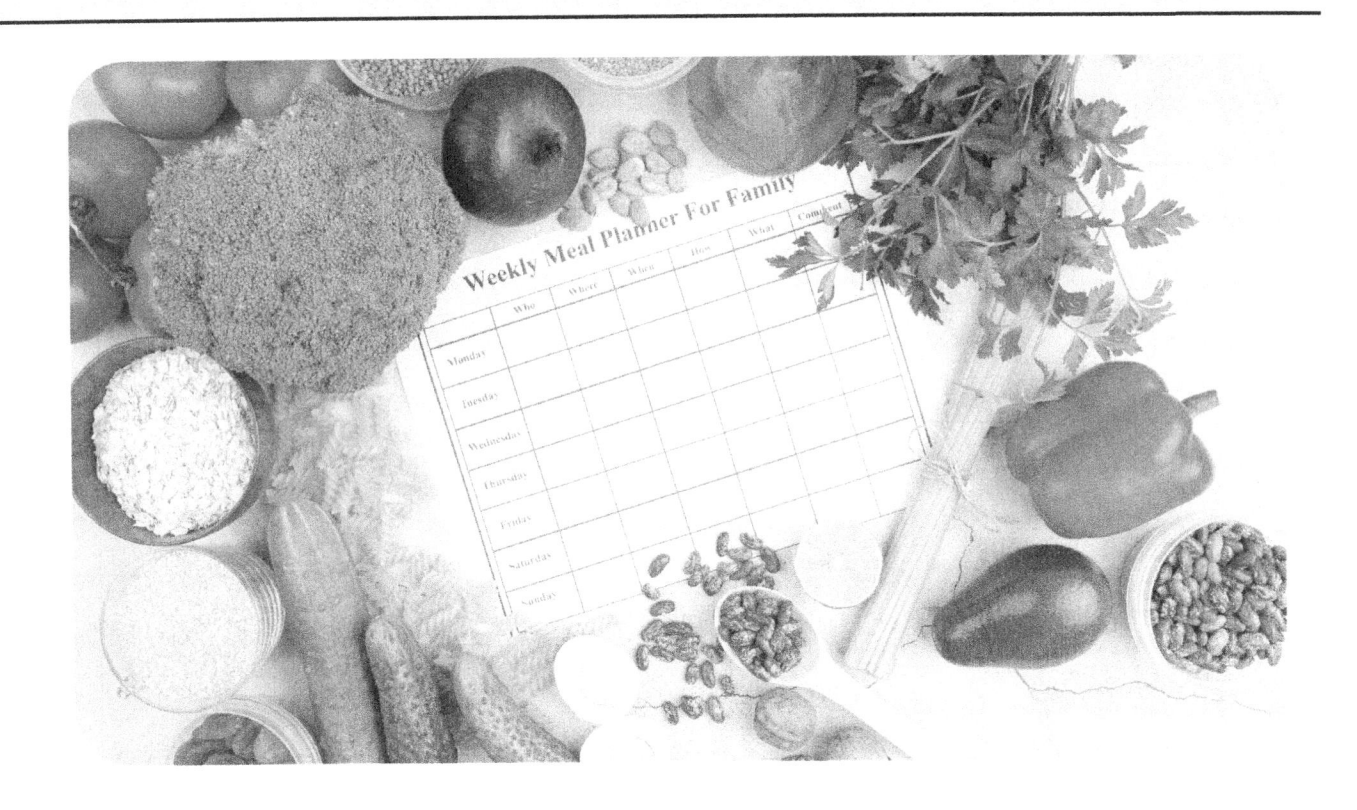

Days	Breakfast	Lunch	Dinner	Dessert
1	CHEESE AND VEGETABLE FRITTATA	PASTA PRIMAVERA	SMOKY HAWAIIAN PORK	PISTACHIO-STUFFED DATES
2	BREAKFAST PIZZA	LEMONY SALMON WITH SPICY ASPARAGUS	HEALTHY PAELLA	MERINGUES WITH STRAWBERRIES, MINT, AND TOASTED COCONUT
3	SPINACH WRAPS	BEEF BRISKET	SWEET AND SOUR CHICKEN WITH RICE	APPLE-BERRY COBBLER
4	QUINOA WITH CINNAMON AND PEACHES	GERMAN POTATO SOUP	CHIPOTLE TACOS	CREPES WITH STRAWBERRIES AND CREAM CHEESE
5	BREAKFAST WRAPS	TOMATO WITH CHEESY EGGPLANT SANDWICHES	BAKED PORK CHOPS	CHOCOLATE "MOUSSE" WITH GREEK YOGURT AND BERRIES
6	VEGETABLE	BEEF AND	PASTA WITH	MASCARPONE

	SHAKE	VEGETABLE STEW	VEGETABLES	AND HONEY FIGS
7	PANCAKES MULTIGRAIN WITH STRAWBERRY SAUCE	QUINOA VEGETABLE SOUP	ZESTY PEPPER BEEF	APRICOT CRISP
8	PORTOBELLO MUSHROOMS FLORENTINE	PARSLEY CHICKPEA BOWLS WITH LEMON	SHISH KABOB	BAKED APPLES WITH ALMONDS
9	CASHEW NUT SHAKE	BEEF AND VEGETABLE KEBABS	PUMPKIN PASTA SAUCE	YOGURT CHEESECAKE
10	BOWL OF GUACAMOLE AND MANGO WITH BLACK BEANS	SALAD WITH BALSAMIC VINAIGRETTE	VEGAN BOWL	CHEDDAR CAKE
11	PEANUT BUTTER OATMEAL	PEPPERED CHEESE WITH STOCKY CAULIFLOWER SOUP	SPICY VEAL ROAST	SWEET POTATO AND PUMPKIN PIE
12	HUMMUS AND DATE BAGEL	HEALTHY MINESTRONE	ITALIAN ROAST	MINT CHOCOLATE DESSERT WITH BANANA
13	CHOCOLATE BANANA OATS	BALSAMIC ROAST CHICKEN	HALIBUT WITH TOMATO SALSA	BAKED APPLES WITH CHERRIES AND ALMONDS
14	CHIA SEED PARFAITS	TOMATO WITH GARLICKY CHIVES	BARBECUED CHICKEN	FRUIT CAKE
15	CURRY TOFU SCRAMBLE	SPINACH BERRY SALAD	YUMMY STEAK BITES	CARROT COOKIES
16	HOMEMADE GRANOLA	SALMON WITH MARINADE	TEFF WITH BROCCOLI PESTO	HOT CHOCOLATE PUDDING
17	BREAKFAST TACOS	QUINOA BOWLS WITH SHRIMP	BARBECUED CHICKEN-SPICY	ROASTED PLUMS WITH WALNUT CRUMBLE
18	BREAKFAST SPLITS	TURKEY KEEMA CURRY	HERB-CRUST COD	APPLE-BERRY COBBLER
19	TOMATO BASIL BRUSCHETTA	CHIPOTLE CHICKEN LUNCH WRAP	HONEY CRUSTED CHICKEN	CHEDDAR CAKE
20	NUTRITIOUS	CHICKEN	HONEY	COOKIE CREAM

	BAGELS	SALAD SANDWICH	CRUSTED CHICKEN	SHAKE
21	SPRING VEGETABLE FRITTATA	POTATO SALAD	WARM BARLEY SALAD WITH SPRING VEGGIES	PISTACHIO-STUFFED DATES
22	BREAKFAST OATMEAL	GARBANZO BEAN CURRY	ZUCCHINI-CHICKPEA BURGERS	BAKED APPLES WITH ALMONDS
23	QUICHE WITH ASPARAGUS, SALMON, AND TOMATO	CARIBBEAN GRILLED PORK	CHICKEN WITH TARRAGON AND LENTILS, PAN-ROASTED	SWEET POTATO AND PUMPKIN PIE
24	CREAMED RICE	HALIBUT WITH LIME AND GINGER	ROASTED SHRIMP AND VEGGIES	APPLE-BERRY COBBLER
25	BANANA OATMEAL CUPS	SMOKED HADDOCK AND SPINACH RYE TOASTS	CHICKEN TENDERS WITH BAGEL SEASONING	ROASTED PLUMS WITH WALNUT CRUMBLE
26	SAUSAGE AND EGG SANDWICH	GRILLED SHRIMP TACOS	CHICKEN WITH LEMON PEPPER AND GARLIC	MERINGUES WITH STRAWBERRIES, MINT, AND TOASTED COCONUT
27	EGG FOO YOUNG	CANNELLINI BEAN PIZZA	SHRIMP AND PINEAPPLE LETTUCE WRAPS	FRUIT CAKE
28	PEANUT BUTTER OATS	LENTILS & RICE	GRILLED SCALLOPS WITH GREMOLATA	CARROT COOKIES
29	TOMATO EGG TART	DEEP, DARK, AND STOUT CHILI	TERIYAKI CHICKEN WITH BLACK RICE AND VEGETABLES	HOT CHOCOLATE PUDDING
30	CRANBERRY HOTCAKES	ORZO, BEAN, AND TUNA SALAD	HONEY-GARLIC CHICKEN THIGHS	BERRIES WITH BALSAMIC VINEGAR

Conclusion

This book is one of the best solutions for safeguarding your heart. Eating healthy and healthy foods is, in fact, the first step to start feeling good. Therefore, as repeated several times, remember that moderate physical activity and a socially active life must also be accompanied by good nutrition.

The benefits that physical activity and human relationships produce in our life have been demonstrated several times. For this reason, you, too, must not give them up.

Finding the right foods for your days and enjoying good company must be your next goal. Finally, remember that there is no single healthy food for your heart; instead, it is the entire diet or diet that you practice every day, in every moment of your life, that benefits your heart and makes it feel suitable and fit.

The heart is, therefore, a very delicate organ that must be safeguarded for the overall health of your body. There are many means and solutions to restore its health, but it is up to you to determine how and when to apply them.

I wish you much joy, health, and prosperity in a life full of beautiful and happy things.

Made in the USA
Monee, IL
08 October 2022